Strength Through Pain

Six Daily Strategies to Live Better
with Chronic Pain

Kevin Bergin

*To all those who persevere in the face of chronic pain,
this book is dedicated to you . . .*

Contents

PART I: FROM THERE TO HERE

PART II: SIX DAILY STRATEGIES

Foreword by Dan John

I read a lot of fitness books. It's a rare week that I don't get a package or PDF filled with the latest and greatest information on how to lean out, bulk up, trim down, and fit in. Some of these books have me going in several directions at once. Rarely do I read a book from someone who has faced discouragement and disappointment.

Strength Through Pain is a remarkable work. Kevin Bergin shares his story of dealing with decades of undiagnosed pain (and the stories of misdiagnosing the issue) that he battled with psoriatic arthritis. Honestly, if he wrote JUST about psoriatic arthritis, I would have been a better coach (and human person!) as I knew very little about this disease. His life story contains dozens of warning signs that Kevin strove to overcome again and again . . . and again.

That's just the beginning of the story. Kevin just didn't let this issue consume him; he overcame it.

If all you learn from the book is the following point, you will be a better person today:

I may wake up stiff every day, but if I go for a walk straight away, I loosen up, and I love walking, so I do that every day, and it's good for your mind and body. I may have limitations, but thanks to arthritis, I've never appreciated my body more than I do now, and I've never been prouder of it.

But there is so much more to this book. Kevin details the key points in successful living. It's nothing shocking:

~ Walk
~ Eat
~ Move
~ Lift
~ Breathe
~ Sleep

I'm sure you KNOW this, but do you do this? It's a question I ask people literally every day of my life. In my experience, only one in 20 people exercise. Of course, only one in 20 floss their teeth appropriately, save enough for a comfortable retirement, or show up when I need help with a house project.

Much of Kevin's work is fundamental. To me, fundamental means: "reasonable, doable, and repeatable". The "doable" part is what Kevin teaches us the best. Personally, his nightly "Do This" list to sleep better is now part of my evening prep for bed.

Strength Through Pain is one of the most fascinating books on fitness, health, longevity, wellness, and body composition I have ever read. It truly is a "one-stop shop" for training advice for the bulk of the population. His life story reminds us that we can all overcome issues and battle towards achieving our goals.

~ Dan John

"You can be anything you want to be . . . But you must be strong first."

~ *Pavel Tsatsouline*

Introduction

I don't really remember anymore what it's like not to feel some sort of pain or discomfort somewhere in my body. It's usually in my hips and spine, though not exclusively. Sometimes it's mild, and other times it's excruciating. Mostly it's somewhere in between. Just how much pain I'm feeling depends on a whole bunch of factors, so there isn't really one thing I can stop doing, or start doing, to cure it. I've been feeling this pain since I was around eighteen, which at the time of writing, was about twenty years ago.

The pain and discomfort are due to psoriatic spondylitis, which is a bit of a mouthful, but put simply, I have arthritis. The psoriatic part references psoriasis – a disease you may have heard of. It manifests as red, itchy, and flaky skin, often on the scalp, but can cover the whole body. Spondylitis refers to the location and means arthritis affects my spine and hips. Up to 30 per cent of people with psoriasis also suffer from psoriatic arthritis. Unfortunately, I have found myself in that 30 per cent.

In the USA, more than one in five adults live with arthritis, which, according to the CDC (Center for Disease Control), makes it a leading cause of disability[1] – that's over 50 million adults. This is also true in Ireland (where I'm from and live), though at a much smaller scale. In the UK, about one in two hundred people are diagnosed with AxSpa,[2] an umbrella term for arthritis that impacts the spine and SI joint (the point where your spine meets your hips). So, there are a lot of us out there living with this type of chronic pain, and if you're reading this, you are likely either living with it yourself or know someone who is.

Unfortunately, there is currently no known cure for psoriatic arthritis. However, various treatment options aim to alleviate symptoms, slow disease progression, and improve the quality of life for those affected. Medical interventions commonly involve a combination of nonsteroidal anti-inflammatory drugs (NSAIDs), disease-modifying antirheumatic drugs (DMARDs), and biologic agents. NSAIDs help manage pain and inflammation, while DMARDs and biologics target the underlying immune system to slow joint damage. While these treatments can be effective, they may also have potential side effects such as gastrointestinal issues, liver toxicity, or increased susceptibility to infections.

Together with medical treatments, lifestyle interventions such as exercise, physical therapy, stress management, and

1 Theis KA, Murphy LB, Guglielmo D, et al. Prevalence of Arthritis and Arthritis-Attributable Activity Limitation — United States, 2016–2018. *MMWR Morb Mortal Wkly Rep* 2021;70:1401–07. DOI: http://dx.doi.org/10.15585/mmwr.mm7040a2
2 NASS. Facts and Figures. https://nass.co.uk/about-as/as-facts-and-figures/

maintaining a healthy weight can also prove extremely effective in treating this and other chronic health conditions. This is important because managing a chronic health condition is not solely your doctor's responsibility. There is a self-management component that is less often talked about but no less important.

I decided to write this book to share my experience of self-managing this chronic condition, hoping others might find my story helpful in their journey with chronic health problems. I also want to share six practical strategies that I learned along the way, which might offer some light amid the desperate feelings that often accompany chronic pain and the knowledge there is no cure – yet. I know the journey isn't an easy one, but in the last 15 years, I have progressed from constant pain through diagnosis to building more strength and mobility than I've ever had in my life. During this time, I learned the things that I want to share with you . . . about how to not only manage the condition but get stronger and more mobile in the process.

I've broken this book down into two parts. In Part I, I'll describe my journey from constant pain, to diagnosis, to now. In part II, I'll share the six strategies you can use to increase your wellbeing, manage pain and live better with arthritis. However, you'll also find that these strategies will work for anyone struggling with any sort of pain and mobility issues or struggling to maintain their health and fitness, irrespective of medical conditions. I've often said that I'm getting a preview of what it's like to be 70 in my thirties; it doesn't feel great, but it is a great teacher.

Lastly, if you're reading this because you're in pain, I urge you to seek help. Don't do what I did – live with a nameless, faceless pain for fifteen years. You don't have to. If you're living with pain and pain gets better with movement but worse with rest, you might be dealing with arthritis. Please, go and get checked out. You will likely need an MRI, but in some cases, an X-ray will do. If you're unhappy with the response you get from your doctor, go get a second opinion. It's much harder to succeed in battle when you don't know what you're fighting. More importantly, it's impossible to accept it.

Part I

From There to Here

My First Flare Up

At eighteen, I went to study Software Engineering at the Institute of Technology Tallaght in Dublin. I went there because I wanted to be a programmer, and it was less than an hour from my house on foot. Most days, I would walk along the main roads toward the building, and if a bus came, I'd hop on. The buses were hard to time, and I'm impatient, so walking wasn't about exercise or anything like that – I just don't like waiting.

One day, as I walked toward college, I saw a bus coming. I didn't feel like walking, so I was happy to see it. However, the bus was rapidly approaching the bus stop, and there was no way I would make it unless I sprinted. So, I did . . . kind of. It was more of an awkward hobble due to the sudden, sharp, intense pain in the right side of my hip. It was as if the socket of that ball and socket joint was lined with sharp spikes.

As I tried to run, the joint stabbed me from the inside, the pain forcing me to keep the leg straight and rigid. I had to avoid creating movement in that hip, so I kept my leg straight and kind of swung it around and in front of me as I moved to avoid heavy contact with the ground. To understand what the movement looks like, try it yourself. Just get up and walk around, but without bending one of your knees. It's not very comfortable or graceful.

I made the bus – out of breath and in quite a bit of pain, but I made it! Actually, I was so out of breath it was embarrassing. I was a little overweight, but my breathlessness was more to do with years of smoking and not exercising. That embarrassment would factor into my future decision to get fit, but I'll come back to that later.

As I boarded the bus and scanned rows of seats for an empty one, I saw a familiar face. It wasn't a friend, but someone that had been in my brother's year in school, so I sat down beside him, and we started talking. It didn't take him long to ask about my awkward, uncoordinated sprint for the bus. I hadn't even thought about the busload of people that had observed me hobbling towards them and how it must have looked incredibly awkward and uncoordinated. My face would have been red with embarrassment at the thought if it hadn't already been bright pink from my lack of fitness.

Anyway, I explained that I had a bad back and that my hip got sore sometimes to the point where just standing on it hurt. And that was that. Just a bad back. I didn't go get checked out or anything, of course. The pain was intermittent, so it came, it sucked, it disappeared, and I forgot about it.

This is my earliest memory of what I now know is a flare-up.

A flare-up is a period where your symptoms become severe.

Sometimes the flare-up lasts a few days, sometimes a few hours, but it's never fun. Also, I'm pretty sure that this wasn't my first flare-up, but it's my earliest memory of one, and the memory is less about the pain and more about the embarrassment I felt. I know I shouldn't have felt ashamed. I was in pain. But our primitive social wiring has strong ways to incentivise not standing out, displaying weakness, or being different.

Diagnosis was around 15 years away at this point.

Something Was Definitely Wrong

Throughout college, I had a few flare-ups, but it never got bad enough to force me to see a doctor. I was living what was probably a pretty typical college lifestyle at the time. I was a regular in the local pub, and when not drinking there, I'd be drinking with friends in someone's house or in my shed (aka The Shed). That's what most Fridays and Saturdays looked like, anyway. The rest of the time, I was in college or sitting on my ass. I wasn't active outside of walking to and from college. No sport, no exercise, nothing like that. I was either sitting at a computer or sitting on a couch.

I also didn't eat very well. Up to and including this point in my life, I didn't consider vegetables real food. My food was mostly beige – potatoes, bread, cheese, ham, chicken, and steak were my staples, washed down with a Coke and followed by chocolate or crisps ("chips" for anyone in the US). I was getting through college just fine, learning to build software, but I wasn't investing in my health or body. To be honest, you can get away with it when you're young.

Young bodies are amazingly resilient. You start to appreciate that fact once you've got around 35 years behind you.

Graduation came in 2007, and I was lucky enough to land a job as a junior software engineer at IBM (large multinational computer hardware and software company, in case you don't know them). My new office was a 40-minute drive away, so I had to learn to drive, and with that, my only form of exercise (walking everywhere) went out the window.

Physically I was doing okay, though. Flare-ups weren't all that common, but something was definitely wrong. I noticed my joints often felt stiff. For example, if I sat on a couch without much back support for too long (which I did all the time), I would have to stand up slowly and audibly. I was in my early twenties but making noises that usually don't accompany movement until your forties or older. Once again, I dismissed this as a bad back. That happens when you spend hours sitting at a computer, right?

At this point, I was still a few years away from going to a doctor and about 12 years away from a diagnosis.

A Change in Lifestyle

I have no idea why I started going for walks in the evening after work – I just did. Post-college, my lifestyle changed. I was at or commuting to/home from work for 10 hours on weekdays. In the evenings, I'd sit around relaxing. Weekends were spent in the pub, so an evening walk just became a way to get out of the house (still my parents' house at this point), away from my siblings, and get some air.

I also had a girlfriend (my now wife), so I was also feeling self-conscious about my body. Actually, to be honest, I've always been self-conscious about it. In my family, I was always the overweight one – although not by 2024 standards, things have changed a lot. But I had tiny little moobs and a bit of a belly. My older brother used to make fun of me for it, which did get to me, but there is one memory that really stands out.

It was probably a Sunday afternoon because the whole family was sitting around the kitchen table having lunch. We usually did that on a Sunday. My younger brother, who was six years old then, was asking about "boobs". It was just innocent curiosity. He was trying to figure out why women have these things on their chests, but men don't, and then pointed at me, saying I looked like I had boobs too.

That one was rough because young kids speak the truth. This wasn't teasing, it was a statement of fact, and it still sticks in my mind thirty years later. My older brother was much more deliberate in his teasing, but that was easier to deal with somehow because he was just being a dick, as older brothers tend to be. But my younger brother's honest observation carved itself into the stone part of my brain, and my chest is still the part of my body that I am most self-conscious of – funny how that works.

Anyway . . . all of that is probably why I started going out for walks in the evening. I'd listen to music and walk a few kilometres, but it took a long time to cover even a modest distance. So, and I hope you're ready for this . . . I thought, *"What if I run instead?"*

I know, a revolutionary idea. But now that I think back, this was around 2007, and there were nowhere near as many people out running for recreation in my little corner of Dublin as there are now. Smartphones were pretty new, and fitness culture wasn't a big thing yet. I didn't really know what I was doing, so like Forrest Gump, I just started running.

My first run was a serious shock to the system. I'd been smoking for over five years at this point. I was probably going through fewer than 10 a day, but it definitely had a significant impact. I'm not sure if lung capacity can be measured in negative numbers, but mine definitely felt like it was a minus something. After a few minutes of running, my lungs gave up on me, though my legs weren't far behind either.

The day after that first run, I felt a pain I'd never felt before. That "day after working some muscles you haven't worked in years" pain. I'd later learn it is known as DOMS, or "delayed onset muscle soreness".

Incidentally, it was around this time that I stopped eating meat, mainly for sustainability reasons, despite not naturally loving vegetables. The global meat production industry just felt wrong to me, and I had read a few books with some scary numbers. I no longer eat a vegetarian diet (I eat fish, but still no other meat), but I do regard going vegetarian to be one of the most important and significant decisions of my life. It was the first time I actually put some thought into the food I was eating, which would prove to be transformative for me.

Did you know . . . Eating more plants has many benefits

Plants are rich in essential nutrients and provide a bunch of the vitamins, minerals, and antioxidants you need for optimal health. By incorporating more plants into your diet, you increase your nutrient intake and ensure your body has the necessary materials for energy production, cell repair, and overall well-being. Leafy greens, colourful vegetables, and fruits are particularly nutrient-dense, offering a variety of vitamins such as vitamin C, vitamin A, and vitamin K, as well as minerals like potassium and magnesium.

Another benefit of consuming more plants lies in their high fibre content, which plays a crucial role in supporting a healthy gut microbiome. Fibre acts as a prebiotic, serving as fuel for beneficial gut bacteria. By nourishing these bacteria, fibre promotes a balanced gut microbiome, linked to improved digestion, enhanced immunity, and even mental health.

In terms of sustainability, shifting towards a plant-based diet can also positively impact the environment. Plant-based foods generally require fewer resources, such as water and land, to produce compared to animal-based products. Livestock agriculture is a major contributor to greenhouse gas emissions and deforestation, while plant-based diets have a lower carbon footprint and can help conserve natural resources. By eating more plants, you can contribute to the preservation of ecosystems, reduction of water usage, and mitigation of climate change.

Remaining time to diagnosis: 10 years or so.

Injury Inclined

After I started running, I noticed pretty quickly that I had a tendency to get injured. At this point, I was twenty-five years old and could run 5–10km, an unthinkable distance from when I first started. I'd do 5km on weekdays and 10km+ on Saturdays. There was no ambition behind it. I wasn't thinking about a future marathon or anything like that. I just liked the feeling. It was the first time in my life that I felt the benefits of physical activity. It was also the kick I needed to stop smoking (though I'd still have a few when drinking, which was also becoming increasingly less frequent).

But something was wrong. My knees were sore, which is pretty typical for runners, but so were my hips and my back. Before long, I just couldn't run anymore. My left knee got bad, and I was starting to wake up with stiff joints in the mornings. The pain of running was rapidly starting to outweigh the benefits.

At this point, I'd love to say I went and spoke to a doctor or physio or anyone about this. I didn't. I had a bad back and, I guess, bad knees too. Oh well. Thankfully that wasn't the end of my growing interest in health and fitness, though, and what follows is my somewhat embarrassing introduction to working out.

Why is it embarrassing? Mainly because the knowledge I've accumulated since means I now know that it was a terrible start to building strength and fitness. Also, I was using pink 2kg dumbbells that my girlfriend bought. Although having said that, I guess it was a good start because I kept going . . . but it wasn't optimal and definitely not advisable for someone with arthritis (which, of course, I still didn't know I had).

The workout program I started with was a series of DVDs (remember those?) from a well-known "celebrity personal trainer" called the "30-day shred". I heard about it from my girlfriend, and its target audience was women who wanted to shred weight, blast abs, and various other things involving fitness industry buzzwords. For me, it was a series of videos I could follow at home that got my heart racing and me breathing heavily in the absence of running.

After a few days on this program, I felt post-workout muscle soreness again, which was interesting. This was the point that I learned that fitness isn't just an all-encompassing generic thing. Before that, I think I just implicitly thought that you're either fit or not. These new workouts came with the realisation that you can be fit for one thing but not another. A long-distance cyclist will be sore if they lift weights for the first time and vice versa.

This is a critically important point. Your body adapts to the stresses that you put on it. It also adapts to the stresses you **don't** put on it.

Your body, both in terms of aesthetics and performance, is a reflection of what you do day to day. A reflection on how you live your life.

I went through that 30-day shred program a few times, and it woke up something inside me. At this point, it was just a flicker, but that spark would eventually become a passion. I started seeking more information and turned to YouTube, where I found a whole bunch of channels with people providing follow-along workouts (all of which are listed in the appendix).

It's hard to put into words just how grateful I am to all of those passionate people that put themselves out there and shared their knowledge and experience for free online. I actually feel a bit emotional just writing this. They have no idea of their impact on my life (and the lives of many others, I'm sure), and in particular:

~ Coach Kozak at HasFIT: https://hasfit.com/
~ Kelli and Daniel at Fitness Blender: https://www.fitnessblender.com/

Two Steps Forward . . . Three Back

These online instructors and classes are where I started. Simple, free home workouts that I could do with a pair of dumbbells and a yoga mat. As I progressed, I became increasingly interested in human physiology and, more importantly, strength. It was never really about aesthetics for me. I wanted to be strong. My desire for strength was possibly a response to my pain, which was getting worse. At this point, my back was constantly sore, but I realised something important. Working out helped it. Temporarily at least. I always felt my best physically after a workout.

I now know that following online workout routines wasn't ideal, considering my undiagnosed underlying condition. These exercise programs are designed for the general population. I'm part of a subset of the general population that needs to approach exercise differently. But they got me to where I needed to be, and for that, I am eternally grateful.

My YouTube curriculum got a bit more advanced after that, thanks to Jeff Cavaliere at Athlean-X (https://athleanx.com). He talks about fitness scientifically, and I voraciously consumed his content. I'd always been interested in science, so his approach to fitness education really clicked for me. I learned all about physiology, as in how the body moves and how it is supposed to move, and with this knowledge in hand, I started to push myself harder to challenge my body. But as my enthusiasm and knowledge increased, my body stopped again and said no, and I was plagued with frequent injuries and enforced downtime. As soon as I started to feel the benefits of working out or got into a routine, my body would start to hurt and tell me to stop.

It's also worth mentioning that there were more changes in my life, the most significant being a new job. In November 2012, I started to work at DIGIT games studio. This was my dream job. I had always wanted to make video games; it was **my why** for studying programming, and now I had the opportunity to do just that. I was working on the server code for our first game, *Kings of the Realm* (the server code is the bit that allows you to play online with other people). Naturally, I was excited and worked damn hard, often putting in 10–12-hour days.

My fitness routine had to accommodate that, so every day, I'd wake up early (before 6 a.m.) stiff as hell and get a workout in before work to help loosen me up. After that came the commute to the office, which was up to an hour on the bus, followed by sitting at a desk all day. All this sitting left me feeling perpetually stiff, so I found myself resorting to over-the-counter anti-inflammatory drugs more and more often.

Did you know . . . Your body hates sitting all day

Sitting for most of the day has become the norm for many people, especially those who work in an office or have a sedentary job. However, prolonged periods of sitting can lead to a host of problems that can affect your physical and mental well-being.

Sitting for a long time can result in poor posture, as the muscles responsible for maintaining an upright position become weak and strained. This can lead to chronic back, neck, and shoulder pain and even spinal misalignment. On top of that, the lack of physical activity associated with sitting all day can contribute to weight gain, muscle degeneration, and a decline in overall fitness.

Another issue caused by prolonged sitting is reduced blood circulation. When sitting, the muscles in the lower body remain static, and blood flow becomes sluggish. This can lead to swollen ankles, varicose veins, and – albeit a worst-case scenario – blood clots. Furthermore, sitting for extended periods is associated with an increased risk of developing chronic conditions such as type 2 diabetes and certain types of cancer, including colon, breast, and endometrial cancer.

Your mental health can also be affected by sitting all day. Sedentary lifestyles have been linked to an increased risk of anxiety and depression and can negatively impact mood, cognitive function, and overall mental well-being.

To mitigate the problems caused by sitting all day, consider incorporating regular movement and breaks into your daily routine. Taking short breaks to stand, stretch, or walk around can help alleviate muscle tension, improve blood circulation, and reduce the risk of associated health issues.

My increasing levels of pain and stiffness did, however, come with a silver lining . . . I finally went to see a doctor and a physio. The downside is that they didn't help.

The physio told me I probably had a bulging disk in my lower back (a common back issue, which, to be fair, has some similar symptoms) and that an MRI would probably just confirm that and, therefore, was a waste of money. Then I went to a doctor and asked her about psoriatic arthritis because I had been reading up on my symptoms online. I knew I had psoriasis and that my symptoms had been worsening, along with the pain, so it seemed logical. She took some blood and told me it was unlikely that I had arthritis. Those tests (incorrectly) confirmed her suspicion.

And so, I was misdiagnosed, which is worse than no diagnosis. I crossed arthritis off the list of possibilities and moved on. There was another silver lining, though. The physio recommended that I try Pilates. It wasn't a silver lining because Pilates is some health and fitness silver bullet or anything like that. It's because it helped me learn more about my body, which was critical for my next step in understanding and dealing with the pain I was living with.

Getting to Know My Body

At this point, I had been doing some home workouts and had done a bit of yoga, all following along to free YouTube videos. I also did a paid program via Athlean-X but couldn't finish because of an injury. Through all this, however, I was constantly learning about what my body could and couldn't do, what made me feel worse vs what made me feel better.

Going to Pilates was a game-changer. It was my first time doing any exercise with an actual in-person instructor. It was weird at first. Mostly because I was a lone thirty-two-year-old male in a sea of strong-cored middle-aged women. I went to that class three times a week while doing my home workouts, and the experience was enlightening. Having someone to explain where my deficiencies were and help me improve was amazing. I know, I know – I'm not going to win a Nobel prize for this insight, but I'd never had any sort of coach before. I had thought that acquiring the knowledge was enough. But **knowledge is not wisdom**. That's what you get from a coach.

I think about the phrase "Practice doesn't make perfect, it makes permanent; perfect practice makes perfect" a lot. Whatever you're trying to learn, it's very difficult to craft a good practice routine on your own. It can be done, but you will save yourself a lot of time and heartache by getting help from others. As I settled into this process of intentional, guided practice, I had another realisation:

You are never not training your body.

Sitting around all day trains your body to sit around all day. Walking trains your body to walk. Lifting weights trains your body to lift weights. But you can also train it poorly (remember, practice makes permanent, not perfect). You might not notice it at first, but the consequences of poor training tend to sneak up slowly and then explode. This is especially true of weight training. You can get away with moving badly for a while, but as the weight you are using increases, so does the risk of serious injury. This is especially true for us arthritics.

Through Pilates, I started to appreciate hands-on instruction, proper movement, and breathing (we will return to breathing later in the book). And through this newfound appreciation for human movement, I stumbled across Callisthenics. The word was new to me and just means "bodyweight training". It's a way to build strength and mobility using only your body. No weights. Just you, your body, and the laws of physics. Think push-ups, pull-ups, squats, etc.

Remember that I was doing Pilates to strengthen my core (I prefer the word "trunk" to describe the midsection, but "core" is perhaps a more familiar term) because I thought it would help with the bulging disk, I thought I had. Callisthenics seemed a great way to help build the strength and mobility needed to fix my back issues.

Diagnosis is still a few years away at this point.

Control Over Tension

I love callisthenics. It is amazing what you can train your body to do with little to no equipment, and I believe it is a skill that would benefit everyone to learn. I can get a great workout no matter where I am or what equipment/facilities are available. And those workouts can build real strength and mastery over your body.

For example, you probably know what a push-up is, and they don't seem too hard, right? But can you do thirty of them without stopping? What if you put your feet up on a chair while you do them? What if you do them with just one arm? There are loads of ways to make a push-up very difficult. You can spend years just working on a single movement. And that is exactly what I did.

This moment was incredibly important because I stopped seeing working out as just following along. I started to really think about my body, what I wanted it to be able to do, and how to progress towards it. I was in charge. But most importantly, I learned that **strength is a skill**.

Being strong isn't all about having big muscles. It's about having control over the tension that you can create in those muscles.

Think about yourself for a minute. Your mind and your body. You could describe that combination as a consciousness piloting the interconnected mess of meat and bones you call your body. The great thing about this point of view is that it implies that you can get better at piloting that body, just like you can get better at driving a car. You can actually improve the control you have over your muscles and your organs. You can make your body perform more efficiently and strengthen it for a greater chance of survival.

Did you know . . . Callisthenics is more than just looking good

Callisthenics, or bodyweight exercises, offer numerous benefits for fitness, health, and well-being. It is an accessible, safe, and effective way to exercise, making it an ideal option for anyone looking to start building strength. Our bodies are designed to move, and callisthenics taps into our natural movement patterns. These exercises mimic our ancestors' daily movements, such as climbing, lifting, and getting up and down from the ground.

One major advantage of callisthenics is that it requires minimal time and equipment. A 20-minute callisthenics workout at home can provide a challenging and effective session, eliminating the need to commute to a gym or invest in expensive equipment. This convenience can lead to increased consistency, which leads to better results.

Another advantage is the reduced risk of injury associated with callisthenics. By working with our body weight rather than heavy weights, we put less strain on our tendons, joints, and muscles. This promotes quicker recovery, allowing for increased workout volume and frequency.

With minimal or no equipment required, you can perform these workouts at home, eliminating the need for gym memberships and reducing associated costs. The time saved from commuting, waiting for machines, or running errands after the gym can be allocated to other things.

Lastly, callisthenics can improve proprioception, the body's internal awareness of its parts. By engaging joints, muscles, ligaments, and connective tissues, callisthenics can enhance body awareness and coordination.

If there was a manual for the human body, it would be huge and incredibly difficult to understand. It all looks so simple on the surface, but once you get beneath the skin, it's a whole other world. This intrigued me. I wanted to be a great pilot.

Thinking back, this realisation wasn't unlike my experience with computers. I started using them as a kid, playing games and messing around, but I was never content with that. I wanted to learn what was going on inside. I wanted to be able to build things. I started making websites at around thirteen years old, back in the late nineties, but that wasn't enough either. I wanted to write computer programs (generally called "apps'" these days). I wanted to make the computer do what I wanted it to do. I wanted to pilot the computer.

As an adult, I found the same curiosity in my body, and callisthenics opened that door. There was a time when I couldn't touch my toes. Actually, I could barely touch my knees. But then, I worked on movement and mobility every day. Now I can place the palms of my hand flat on the ground from a standing position without bending my knees. This was unimaginable to me ten years ago. Eventually, I got strong and skilled enough to do that one-armed push-up—one-legged squats too. It took ages, but I kept chipping away and got the results. There's a life lesson buried in there:

Trust the process, and the results will take care of themselves.

Building Strength

I worked towards a one-armed push-up for months, gradually progressing from a regular push-up. Want to know what happened on the day I hit my first one?

Nothing. I did it and had a moment of childlike excitement, that feeling where your body is brimming with energy, and you need to punch the air or jump up and down just to let it out, and then, with a big smile on my face, I went about my day. Nothing changed. The world didn't stop to celebrate my achievement. It was just another fleeting moment in time.

That's the interesting thing about a goal. Nothing really changes when you hit it. There's a moment, or maybe a couple of days, where you feel accomplished and proud, but it's almost immediately followed by the question, *"What now?"*

It seems to me that the process is where the value is. That's where the lessons are learned, and the change happens. I've hit a few personal and professional goals over the years, and it's always the same. I think that's because worthwhile goals take time – a long time. While striving to reach them, you are constantly progressing, which is why achieving the goal doesn't feel like a big leap or anything like that. It's just another day of working.

It's kind of like growing your hair. If you have short hair and don't cut it for a year, it will, of course, grow. You look at yourself in the mirror every day and grow accustomed to whatever is looking back at you. Over time you forget what "short-haired you" looked like as you slowly morph into "long-haired you". Then a day comes when you have long hair and can tie it up or do whatever you want to do with it. To you, it doesn't feel like all that much has changed. However, if someone saw you on day one of your hair growth but didn't see you for the following year, their mental image of your appearance would be immediately shattered. To them, it would be a shock, a huge change, but to you, it's a gradual, unnoticeable change.

Anyway, I loved callisthenics and was achieving my strength and fitness goals, but naturally, I was getting a bit bored. I wanted to explore something else, and that's when I landed on kettlebells, thanks to the work of Pavel Tsatsouline.

Did you know ... Kettlebells were once a tool for measuring grain

The kettlebell is a popular fitness tool, but its origins can be traced back to Russia in the 18th century when they were used as counterweights in markets to measure grains. Over time, people began to recognise their potential as a tool for physical training and started incorporating them into their exercise routines.

In the late 19th century, Russian strongmen and athletes utilised kettlebells to develop strength and power. The popularity of kettlebell training grew, becoming a fundamental part of physical education and military training in Russia. The Russian military, in particular, adopted kettlebell exercises to enhance soldiers' overall physical fitness and combat readiness.

Kettlebell training methods and techniques were refined and systematised by the Russian physician Vladislav Kraevsky. He developed a comprehensive training system known as Girevoy Sport, which involved repetitive kettlebell movements for endurance and strength. This marked the formalisation of kettlebell training as a sport.

In the 20th century, kettlebells gained international recognition and spread beyond Russia. In the 1980s, Russian kettlebell techniques were introduced to the United States by Pavel Tsatsouline, a former Soviet Special Forces physical training instructor. Tsatsouline popularised kettlebell training in the West through his books, workshops, and certifications. The kettlebell became a staple tool in the fitness industry, with trainers and enthusiasts embracing its versatility and effectiveness for functional training.

Today, kettlebell training has become a mainstream fitness trend worldwide. It is utilised by athletes, strength and conditioning coaches, and fitness enthusiasts of all levels. Kettlebells offer a unique combination of strength, cardio, and flexibility training, providing a full-body workout.

Pavel Tsatsouline is a strength coach that specialises in kettlebell training. He credits himself as introducing Kettlebells to the West, having been a staple of Russian strength training for decades.

A kettlebell is simply a cast iron ball with a handle attached, and Pavel's books and videos got me interested in them. You can, it turns out, do a lot with a single kettlebell. They are an incredibly useful tool for building strength and endurance. They're probably not the **best** gym kit for building strength since you're limited in how heavy you can get, but they are a great addition to any workout routine.

The kettlebell swing is the signature exercise and involves swinging the bell between your legs and up to about chest height. This simple movement helps strengthen your core, glutes, back, and hamstrings – all critical for daily movement and power. My SI joint (where the spine meets the hips) is a problem for me, and I've found that this movement helps keep it moving smoothly. If I'm sore, I know doing a few swings will bring instant relief.

However, for me, the real advantage of a kettlebell is that it takes up basically no space in your home, and it covers some gaps of pure callisthenics. So, between your body and your bell, you can make a lot of progress. I have 10-minute workouts with a single bell that will leave my muscles burning and my breath nowhere to be found.

Over the years, I have accumulated nine kettlebells (1 * 8kg, 2 * 16kg, 2 * 24kg, 2 * 32kg, 1 * 40kg), and I'm sure I will have more in the future. That selection of weights combined with a 3ft x 6ft space in my spare bedroom has been my home gym for years. You don't even need that much. One appropriately weighted kettlebell (likely 16kg for women, 24kg for men) and a small amount of floor space is all you need to build a solid base of strength and fitness, or day-to-day strength. The kind of strength that makes you a real asset to friends that are moving house or need some help clearing out a garden.

Pavel reinforced in me the idea that **strength is a skill**. So, what does that really mean? It means that strength is not just about big muscles; it is a skill you learn, like learning to write or play guitar. In fact, you can get a lot stronger without building any muscle at all. You just need to teach your brain and muscles to operate more efficiently.

It is the same as when you want your car to go faster; you could give it a bigger engine **or** make the engine it already has run more efficiently. The latter is what strength training does. You are improving the connection between your brain and muscles (neuromuscular connection). Essentially strength training makes it so that the electrical signals that get sent to your muscles when they need to do work are amplified. If you want to see real strength, watch some Olympic lifters on YouTube. They, for the most part, don't look like giant, ripped bodybuilders, but they tend to be a lot stronger.

Breathing Through Pain

Another important idea I took away from Pavel, and working with kettlebells, was about breathing. Specifically, "power breathing". This technique lets you sync your breath with your movement to maximise power output. Basically, breathe out on the hard part and make it a short sharp breath.

I had previously learned to better control my breath through Pilates, which was focused on breathing to facilitate better movement. That, combined with this power breathing, is, I think, one of the top two, if not the most important thing I've learned during this journey. It has gotten me through many "arthritis days", as I call them. Those days when your arthritis is really acting the prick.

There are a couple of things to cover here. One is bracing. The other is power and mobility.

Let's start with bracing.

If you watch a powerlifter lifting heavy weights, you will notice that they will take a deep breath right down into their belly before doing a big lift. This creates a cushion of air in their abdomen and acts as a support for their spine.

Try it now. Stand up and take a deep breath right down deep into your belly and hold it. But don't just hold it; squeeze it. Feel the tension ripple out from your abdomen to the rest of your body. Squeeze your fists too, and your glutes. Your body should feel tight, and it should feel strong.

I often do this when standing up from a seat if I feel particularly sore. I will breathe into my belly, hold, and then release as I stand up. If my joints are sore, especially my lower back or hips, this relieves a lot of pressure. It's like my muscles step in and say to my joints, "We got this!"

There's an important detail here, though. As you breathe out, you don't want to let the air and tension flop out of your body. You need to control it. The easiest way to do this is to hiss. Literally. Make a hissing sound. Exhale sharply but keep the passage of air narrow. This is what hissing does for you. As you hiss the air out, you can feel that the tension is still there, but some energy is freed up for other things, like movement. This is where the power is.

If you've ever watched a boxing match, you've seen this in action. Ever notice how when a boxer throws a punch, it's accompanied by a kind of sharp hissing sound? They breathe sharply out of their nose as they strike.

As an analogy, think about a balloon. When it's inflated, you can feel the tension. If you puncture it with a pin, the balloon flops to the ground with a bang. However, if you release the balloon's valve and let go, it will fly around the room. The tension dissipates, but it's transformed into movement.

Tension turns to energy. This is how I picture what is going on inside my body. I inflate a balloon inside me as I breathe in, and then as I breathe out, I convert that tension to energy. All that being said, learning to breathe isn't all about creating tension.

Breathing can help you really step into your own body.

Try this exercise to see this for yourself.

Stand up and try to touch your toes. Keep your legs straight and bend over as far as you can. Even if it's just to your knees. Once you reach your limit, breathe in. A big belly breath if you can manage it. Then breathe out, slow and controlled, but with the hiss. As you breathe out, try to stretch further. I'm certain you'll find a bit more range.

Learning about proper breathing techniques was huge for me. Of all the things I've learned about my body, this genuinely stands out as one of the most important for helping me deal with arthritis and the associated pain. Though at this point, I still didn't know I had arthritis. I just knew it helped me be stronger, move better and work through the pain. We're getting close now, though, only two years away from a diagnosis. I was learning more about my body each day and was hungry to learn more.

Nourishing Body and Mind

In 2018, I decided to train as a personal trainer. Not because I was looking for a career change but because I wanted to learn all I could about my body and how to train it. So, I signed up for a six-month part-time course. It was a combination of theory and practical lessons in a gym. We learned about anatomy and physiology, putting together exercise programs, etc., and spent time on the gym floor with coaches learning how to move and coach movements.

It was sometimes frustrating because I couldn't do some of the movements. I was just in too much pain. This is partly because I had a whole new host of equipment and movements to work with, so my body had some adaptation to do. I find that when I throw too many new things at my body, I tend to pay the price. But it was worth it, and by the end, I felt confident that I could construct a good path forward for myself. A path that would help me build strength, move better, and eventually get over this damn bulging disk!

When I finished that course, I started doing something I have continued to this day – taking notes. I buy a diary every year, and every day I write down whatever exercises I have done. Every workout, every rest day, every short walk, and every long hike for the last five years are all meticulously tracked in my diaries. These diaries are the most important piece of fitness equipment I own. And with five years of history already recorded, do you think I want to break that chain? Of course not. Buying a new diary each year is a ritual at this point. It's also nice to look back and see my progress. The strength gains have been significant.

With my newfound coaching knowledge and diaries tracking my progress, my workouts became an organised combination of Pilates, yoga, kettlebells, and callisthenics. I was focused on mobility, strength, and power. Notice that I've yet to mention anything about body composition. During this journey, my body changed, I built muscle and lost body fat, but that was just a side effect. I was trying to feel good and, more importantly, feel strong.

Feeling healthy and strong is a much better motivation and more sustainable than aesthetic goals.

Speaking of body composition, the personal training course also covered diet and nutrition, and during this whole journey through fitness, I found that my interest in food and nutrition also grew. The two are inextricably linked. You need to be eating well to recover from your workouts and make progress in terms of strength and work capacity.

I mentioned already that I used to be a vegetarian (now a pescetarian), a decision driven mostly by the ecological and moral disgrace of factory farming. I even went vegan for a year, though that wasn't sustainable, and I felt worse physically during that period. That might not be true for everyone, but it was for me. I had digestive issues, which I've found come with increased arthritic pain. Your mileage may vary.

The important point is that I have learned over the years that diet plays a huge role in my experience with arthritis. If I eat like crap, I feel like crap. If I eat a lot of sugar, I will be sore the next day. If I eat to the point of feeling bloated, I will be sore. If I'm constipated, I'm generally also sore. So, like my decision to train as a personal trainer to better understand my body and how to train it, I decided to train as a nutrition coach.

In 2018, after receiving my personal training certification, I signed up for a Precision Nutrition course. This was an industry-leading course in nutrition coaching. I had already covered nutrition in the personal training course, but this took it to the next level.

One of the challenges around diet and nutrition is that there is a lot of information out there and many people trying to sell you all sorts of products. Some people eat nothing but raw meat, there are vegans, and there is everything in between. Some people will tell you that carbs are the work of the devil, and others will say that reducing the amount of protein and fat you eat is the secret to a long life.

Precision Nutrition cuts through all that crap and gives sensible, balanced information. Their concern is helping people understand how to make long-term sustainable positive changes around diet. It was incredibly useful as I tend to go to extremes.

At this point, my diet was generally pretty clean. I tried to follow the Precision Nutrition standard, which was that each meal should consist roughly of the following:

- ~ A palm-sized piece of protein (meat, fish, eggs, tofu, etc.)
- ~ A fist-sized portion of vegetables
- ~ A cupped hands portion of carbs (bread, pasta, grains, etc.)
- ~ A thumb-sized piece of fat
- ~ Drink plenty of water throughout the day and in-between meals.

I love this approach because it is easy to internalise and customise to your needs and will work for most people. But something else had a huge impact on me from a diet and nutrition point of view... and that was simply not eating.

It turns out that fasting has many benefits for the human body. I first tried it in 2019 when the intermittent fasting craze hit. The idea is to eat for some set period throughout the day, say 8 hours, and then fast for the rest. I tried it (16 hours of fasting each day) and had great results. I generally feel my best, in terms of arthritis symptoms, when I haven't eaten in 12+ hours. Now, I hope it goes without saying that you still need to nourish your body with good food while doing this. You are not starving yourself; you are just giving your body's digestive system a much-needed rest.

Did you know . . . Fasting has a host of health benefits

I find that I feel great when I fast. This is becoming more popular, and you'll find plenty of books and on-line resources. I often fast for 16 hours out of 24 hours, but even a 12-hour (8 p.m. to 8 a.m., for example, has benefits.

Some of those benefits include:

- **Blood sugar control:** Fasting has been shown to improve blood sugar control and insulin resistance.

- **Inflammation reduction:** Chronic inflammation is associated with a bunch of health conditions. Studies have found that fasting can decrease inflammation markers, such as C-reactive protein.

- **Heart health improvement:** Fasting has shown potential to improve heart health by reducing total cholesterol, blood pressure, and triglyceride levels. It may lower the risk of coronary artery disease and diabetes, both major risk factors for heart disease.

- **Brain function enhancement:** Animal studies suggest fasting improves brain function and structure. It may also protect against neurodegenerative disorders like Alzheimer's and Parkinson's by increasing nerve cell synthesis and relieving inflammation.

- **Weight loss support:** Fasting can aid in weight loss as your calorie intake tends to be reduced.

Advisory: While fasting can offer many health benefits, it is essential to approach it cautiously and consult with a healthcare professional, especially if you have a specific medical condition, pregnant, breastfeeding, underweight or have other dietary needs.

At this point, I had all the information I needed to create training programs and a healthy balanced diet plan. I should also point out that I've never been on a diet. That word is pretty loaded. I use the word 'diet' in the sense that everyone has a diet. It's whatever you eat day to day. I don't like the idea of short-term or crash diets. Generally, when it comes to exercise and eating, I think if you can't do it for the next ten years, then what's the point? There are no hacks here.

The Pain Explained . . . Finally

Finally, we've made it. Diagnosis – albeit 15 years later.

It was 2019, and I was sick of everything. Of being sore all the time. Of not being able to sleep due to pain. Of limping around despite being in good physical shape. So I decided to go to a different physio. He ran me through some movement drills and was impressed with the flexibility and strength I had built up. So much so that his immediate reaction was, "You need to see a rheumatologist." So I did. I found a doctor specialising in spondylitis, and he had me go for an MRI (magnetic resonance imaging) scan immediately, which confirmed inflammation in my spine and SI joint.

That's what this condition is – chronic inflammation. Which, by the way, isn't just painful but comes with a whole host of other problems, such as the increased risk of:

~ Cancer
~ Diabetes
~ Neurological diseases
~ Cardiovascular diseases
~ Alzheimer's disease

Despite that, I actually felt pretty good after the diagnosis. The monster had a name, which made it a lot easier to fight it. But that mindset is also dangerous. This disease is currently incurable, so it's important to avoid thinking that you have control over it. You don't. But if you think you do, you naturally blame yourself for it, and it's all too easy to start thinking, *"Oh, I'm sore today. That must be because I did X."* That can result in a lot of mental strain.

And, in fact, it did. The two years following diagnosis were pretty rough regarding my mental health. It's hard to feel any sort of positive emotion about the future when you know that pain is always going to be there. And that's where I learned my next lesson . . .

Acceptance.

It is what it is. If you don't accept your reality, whatever it may be, you'll probably have a bad time. At this point, reading up on Stoicism really helped. Stoicism is a school of thought that focuses on the idea that the only thing you can control is your reaction to the things happening around you.

Did you know . . . Sometimes the answer lies in looking back

Stoicism is an ancient philosophy that originated in ancient Greece around the 3rd century BCE. It was developed by Zeno of Citium and later expanded upon by notable philosophers such as Epictetus and Marcus Aurelius. Stoicism aims to teach you how to live a virtuous and fulfilled life by focusing on personal ethics, resilience in the face of adversity, and accepting the things you cannot control.

The Stoics believed that the key to happiness and tranquillity lies in understanding and aligning yourself with the universe's natural order. They emphasised the importance of developing self-discipline, self-control, and moral virtue, which they believed were the foundations of a good life. Stoicism encourages you to focus on the present moment, accept things as they are, and not be disturbed by external events or circumstances beyond your control.

Stoicism gained popularity throughout the Roman Empire and influenced statesmen, philosophers, and emperors. It has continued to have a lasting impact on Western philosophy and has experienced a resurgence in modern times. Its teachings have been integrated into various fields, including psychology, self-help, and personal development, as Stoic principles provide practical guidance for dealing with life's challenges and finding inner peace.

The question for me now was, what do I do **despite** this shitty disease? My thoughts ran something like this: "I won't ever be able to run a marathon, I know that - but you know what, I've built enough strength to be able to press half my own body weight over my head, with one arm. How do you like that arthritis?"

I may wake up stiff every day, but if I go for a walk straight away, I loosen up, and I love walking, so I do that every day, and it's good for your mind and body. I may have limitations, but thanks to arthritis, I've never appreciated my body more than I do now, and I've never been prouder of it.

I should mention that when I was diagnosed, the first thing the rheumatologist did was try to put me on some pretty heavy drugs. A new class of drugs called "biologics", which are made from living organisms and can effectively reduce chronic inflammation and involve regular self-administered injections. However, these drugs come with an extensive list of side effects as they can reduce the function of your immune system, leading to increased risk of:

~ Cancer
~ Serious infections, including TB, and infections caused by viruses, fungi, or bacteria.
~ Allergic reactions
~ Nervous system problems
~ Blood problems (decreased blood cells that help fight infections or stop bleeding)
~ Heart failure (new or worsening)
~ Immune reactions, including a lupus-like syndrome
~ Liver problems
~ Psoriasis (new or worsening)

I decided not to take the drug, but I want to be clear that I am not advocating against taking this or any other class of prescription drug that has been recommended by your medical professional. They can be life-changing for people that are really suffering. I appreciate that I am actually doing pretty well and that this disease is far more debilitating for many people out there than it is for me. I do recommend that you research any prescribed drugs so you can make an informed decision.

However, I consider them an absolute last resort rather than a first port of call. I may take them someday, but not now. I want to try other things first. I want to try everything first. This isn't a drug that you can just stop taking. Taking it would mean I have a hard dependency on a pharmaceutical company... and I'm sorry, but I just don't trust them, and I don't want to rely on them and the supply chain that gets the drug into my hands.

How It Feels

So, what does arthritis actually feel like?

This is a difficult question to answer. Pain is interesting. You can try and describe it, but it's different for everyone. Even pain that appears to be the same type will feel different to different people. For example, I have quite a few tattoos, many in sensitive places (around the knees, near the armpits). I generally sit quite well for tattoos. It's painful, sure, but I can deal with it. However, I know some people that couldn't go through it without having their skin numbed. I know others that gave up halfway through getting their first tattoo.

When it comes to arthritis, it's not one type of pain that I feel. The pain tends to move around my body, usually focused on one area at any given time, though this isn't true for everyone. I've spoken to others that feel the effect in multiple joints simultaneously.

Did you know . . . Pain isn't just a physical thing

External factors play a significant role in the perception and experience of pain. One crucial factor that can amplify the sensation of pain is the lack of quality sleep. When you haven't slept well, your threshold for pain tends to decrease, and even minor discomfort can become magnified. Sleep deprivation not only affects the body's ability to cope with pain but also disrupts the normal functioning of the central nervous system, heightening pain sensitivity. The body's natural pain-modulating mechanisms may become compromised, making the pain feel more intense and challenging to manage.

Living through a particularly stressful period can also contribute to an exacerbated experience of pain. Stress, whether related to work, relationships, or personal circumstances, can intensify pain perception. The body's stress response triggers the release of stress hormones, such as cortisol, which can heighten pain sensitivity. Stress often leads to muscle tension and increased inflammation, further amplifying pain signals. During stressful times, you may also experience heightened anxiety and emotional distress, which can intensify the emotional component of pain. This emotional aspect should not be overlooked, as it can significantly impact the overall experience and perception of pain.

Recognising the emotional component of pain is crucial for understanding its complexity. Pain is not solely a physical sensation but also a subjective experience influenced by your emotional state. Anxiety, fear, depression, and distress can all significantly magnify the perceived intensity of pain. The brain processes pain signals in conjunction with emotional and cognitive factors, forming a complex interplay that shapes the overall pain experience. Emotional distress can increase the focus on pain, leading to a heightened awareness of discomfort and a reduced ability to cope effectively.

When assessing and managing pain, it's important to consider the broader context of your life. Understanding external factors such as sleep quality, stress levels, and emotional well-being can provide valuable insights into your experience of pain.

I mostly feel pain distinctly in the following areas:

~   Lower back
~   Hips (it swaps between the left and right side)
~   The big toe on my right foot
~   My ribs
~   My left wrist
~   The back left-hand side of my ribcage
~   My upper back

I feel it elsewhere too, but these areas are the most predominant. And each one is a little bit different.

When it comes to my spine, I like to imagine a spine made of aluminium cans. Each can is full, pressurised, and represents a single vertebra. Between each can is a spongy disc, just like a regular spine. Now, if that is a normal spine, then mine looks a little different. Like someone has opened, emptied, and slightly crushed and twisted each of my aluminium vertebrae. If you take a can and grip the top and bottom and then twist it and crush it a little, it will compress, and the edges will become jagged. They will no longer be uniform. As the spine moves around, the sharp jagged edges dig into the surrounding tissue. They have no structural integrity. The whole thing feels weak, as if it could collapse at any moment. The spongy bits between them have also degraded so that the cans are rubbing against each other.

In my lower back, the pain can be enough to just stop me in my tracks. Like, sometimes I go to stand up and just stop halfway, maybe sit back down. It's as if one of the cans is about to tear. It's a pain that I've also described as being like a "Chinese burn" being performed on your spine (A "Chinese burn" is a schoolyard trick, something kids used to do when I was in school. You grab someone's forearm with both your hands and twist in opposite directions. It feels like your skin will tear, and it feels horrible). This pain is usually felt during some sort of transition, from sitting to standing or from standing to sitting. If you watch me stand up, you will notice that I usually sit forward to the edge of the chair, get my arms involved and assume perfect squat form. I don't just stand up.

In my upper back, the feeling is similar but less severe. The cans are a little less crushed. The pain is more like pressure. It's blunt rather than sharp. It makes me feel like I have a limited range of motion, as though I can't extend that part of my spine (bend it backwards). It is less debilitating than the lower back – but it's still pretty unpleasant.

In my wrist and big toe, I have a similar sort of feeling. With inflammatory arthritis, your joints get inflamed, and the body can respond by laying down new bone. This can mean that the space between your joints is shrinking, and new bone is being created. This is what is going on in my wrist and toe. I can feel a bump in each. On my toe, it's visible, and it can't move as much as it should be able to. I can bend my left big toe back normally, but my right one quickly hits a wall. This pain is a dull, pressure kind of pain. You can simulate this by gripping the middle and index finger of your bad hand with your good hand and squeezing hard. Squeeze hard enough so that you can feel the finger joints pressing against each other. It's not nice.

The rib pain was a surprise to me. I had never really considered they were joints too. What sucks about pain here is that it makes breathing hard and painful. Like the lower back, it can be a sharp and stabbing pain. If I'm feeling sore here and take a big deep breath, one that really expands my ribcage, I sometimes feel a sharp pain that forces an exhale, kind of like a punch in the stomach. In fact, I've been talking before, and mid-sentence made a weird noise, like *"hhunngggghhh"*, as though my ribs said, *"Nope, you're done talking."* This one is bad for sleep too. I've woken myself up before by breathing too heavily and triggering this one. It flares up if I sit and lean to the side, putting pressure on the ribcage.

And finally, the hips. I've saved the worst for last. The place where I felt that first flare-up.

Ever stood on a piece of Lego? Imagine that instead of standing on it, it is inside your hip joint. And if you move your leg in certain ways, the Lego gets wedged between the leg bone and the hip bone and just kind of grinds around in there. It's sharp and painful, and you know it's just sitting there . . . waiting. You can get in a certain position where it's not sore, but it's still lurking. Waiting for you to make one wrong move.

When this joint gets bad, it's really bad. Sitting is uncomfortable, standing is uncomfortable, and lying down is uncomfortable. This pain and immobility mean I also walk with a limp when it is bad, and it's when the disease feels most externally visible to me. It's just a bad time. I wouldn't recommend it. A bad hip day will usually result in me taking an anti-inflammatory, which I generally try to avoid as much as possible.

It's also worth mentioning the emotional weight of all of this. It's exhausting. If you've been sore for a few days, you can become pretty irritable and tired, too, because you probably haven't slept well. If you're not careful, a real sense of nihilism and depressive moods can creep in. Everything can just feel shit and pointless. For me, it's not that I'd actively want to die. I'd just care less about living. This can really start to drag you down if you let it, and that is why I put so much effort these days into cultivating strength, both mental and physical.

Did you know . . . Gratitude practice can be healing

Gratitude is a powerful emotion that can benefit your overall well-being and relationships. When we practice gratitude regularly, we cultivate a positive mindset and shift our focus towards acknowledging and appreciating the good things in our lives. One of the significant benefits of gratitude is its impact on our mental health. Expressing gratitude has been shown to reduce stress, anxiety, and depression. It allows us to reframe our thoughts and find positives in difficult situations, fostering a sense of optimism and hope.

On top of that, gratitude has physical health benefits as well. Research has shown that practising gratitude can reduce symptoms of pain and inflammation.[3] By reducing stress and promoting relaxation, gratitude indirectly supports our physical well-being. When we cultivate gratitude, we tend to engage in healthier behaviours and consciously prioritise self-care. This can include maintaining regular exercise routines, practising mindfulness, and adopting healthier eating habits, all contributing to overall wellness.

This sort of practice is not new, either. It's what a Christian would call "prayer", a quiet, reflective period where you thank God for all you have and ask that those you care about find comfort and peace. A Buddhist might call it "loving-kindness meditation". Ancient Assyrians and Babylonians, all the way back in 3000 BCE, used hymns and litanies to express gratitude to their gods.

Whatever the name and form of this gratitude, practices like this rarely stick around for centuries unless

3 Carson JW, Keefe FJ, Lynch TR, et al. Loving-Kindness Meditation for Chronic Low Back Pain: Results from a Pilot Trial. Journal of Holistic Nursing. 2005;23(3):287-304. doi:10.1177/0898010105277651

there is some benefit, regardless of whether that benefit is scientifically proven.

Thankfully, I don't feel the extremes of these most days. I'm managing it pretty well through a combination of various things that I will detail in the next section. Though I should say I feel hip and lower back pain right now as I write this. I actually waited until I was feeling some pain to write this section so that I could write what I felt as I felt it. Interestingly, writing it all out like this makes me feel grateful that I don't feel these symptoms so severely most of the time and that there is a lot I can do in the face of this disease. There are many people out there that who are a lot worse off than I am, and I really am lucky that I've been able to do what I can despite all this.

The Things That Help

Since that first flare-up after running for the bus, I've learned much about this disease and how to better live with it. I'm the strongest I've ever been physically . . . and I've honed six strategies that help me manage arthritis.

So, what do I do? In short:

~ Walk
~ Eat
~ Move
~ Lift
~ Breathe
~ Sleep

Of course, what works for me and suits my life, and my schedule may not work for anyone else. You should at least think about each of these strategies, but how you implement them will be uniquely you. The whole point of walking through this journey was to highlight my discovery process. I believe that everyone needs to go through that process and find what really works for them.

Everything I write here is meant to serve as inspiration, not a ruleset.

I'll share more about these strategies in Part II, but here's the overview.

Walk

I truly believe that walking should be considered a form of medicine. Everyone seems to intuitively understand that you need to walk a dog regularly, but most don't apply the same logic to themselves.

Our bodies are built for walking. I even find walking in terrible weather beneficial in its own way, if only so you appreciate the nice days more. Short relaxing walks are restorative, and being in nature is great for your mental health (Japanese therapists have even been known to prescribe patients *shinrin yoku* or forest bathing – simply being among the trees.)

I walk every day, usually first thing in the morning. Just a 20-minute walk. On days I'm not doing a heavy workout, I'll usually extend the walk to 40–60 minutes. I also like hiking once a week if I can.

Eat

Diet is huge for me. In fact, I would go as far as to say that I am allergic to sugar. If I eat a lot of sugar, I will be sore the following day. Eating a lot of fibre, on the other hand, really seems to help. I once did an elimination diet where I only ate sweet potatoes, eggs, leafy greens, nuts, and eggs for a month. It felt like my arthritis had just disappeared. Now, it was completely unsustainable, but it taught me that diet is key and that I must stay on top of it. Also, I feel at my best physically when I have done a fast. And I feel much better when I don't eat at least three hours before bed.

I eat a lot of vegetables, eggs, and fish, but no other meat. I avoid sugar as much as possible. I only drink water and herbal tea. In terms of supplementation, I take an all-in-one vitamin supplement and krill oil daily.

Move

This is all about stretching and mobility and is critical for me. My joints are trying to seize up and fuse together every day. I just don't let them. These days I see a mobility specialist and am very mobile and flexible, all things considered. If you looked at me doing this stuff, you wouldn't believe I have an arthritic spine! I start every day with a mobility and stretching routine and end every day with some stretching and light movement, along with dedicated mobility classes and yoga.

Lift

Lift weights – but do it properly. I need my muscles to be strong to support my shitty joints. I believe that everyone should lift weights. You may have different limitations to me but try and find a way to do some resistance training. The health benefits are immense, both physically and mentally.

I think the most significant thing that lifting weights did for me was to teach me that if I focus on something and apply consistent effort, I will get better and achieve my goals. And if me and my arthritic spine can do it, you most likely can too.

I lift at least three times a week. I call these my "heavy days". Then I'll also do two lighter days, where I'm lifting or using my body weight but trying not to strain my body too much.

Breathe

Along with the power breathing and meditative breathing I mentioned earlier, I learned about Wim Hof in 2020 and have been doing his breathing exercises ever since. His breathing method, in particular, really helps me fall asleep if I do it before bed and reduces anxiety if I'm having an "arthritis day".

I also start each day with breathing exercises and try to be conscious of my breath throughout the day. I have a breathing-related mantra that I try to keep in the back of my mind at all times: "Breathe through your nose and into your belly. Light and slow."

Sleep

Sleep is hard for me. Sitting or lying still breeds stiffness, and sleep involves mostly lying still. Tossing and turning can be painful if I'm stiff, which tends to wake me up. But sleep is important. Really important. It's when your body recovers from whatever stresses have been placed on it during the day, both mentally and physically.

I try to follow good sleep practices to minimise the disruption, but I often fail. I've found that not doing something (e.g. not eating before bed) can be a lot harder than doing something (e.g. going for a walk), which is counterintuitive but holds true for me.

In Part II, we'll dive deeper into how you can use these six strategies to thrive despite arthritis. These six daily habits or strategies can change how you see the world and, for the most part, won't require spending any money. Just time. And, at the end of the day, the only thing any of us has is time, so it's probably worth considering how you spend it and the impact that today's investment has on your future return.

Part II

Six Daily Strategies

1. Walk

> *"Me thinks that the moment my legs begin to move, my thoughts begin to flow."*
>
> ~ Henry David Thoreau (American writer and philosopher)

Movement Is Medicine

This isn't homework; it's an opportunity.

I would love it if we celebrated walking in adulthood as we do when we watch our children take their first steps. It's a momentous occasion. Parents, relations, and siblings sit around, shout encouragement, and beam with pride as a tiny little human takes their first steps. After that, we accept this daily physical miracle without applause – it's normal. It's such an innate thing, so natural for our bodies, that we immediately take it for granted. However, I acknowledge that not everyone can walk. If you, for whatever reason, cannot, consider everything in this section to be about "moving" through the world and spending more time outside in nature if possible.

Movement Matters

Some anthropologists estimate that our ancestors became bipedal around six million years ago, so we've been walking for a long time, and our bodies have gotten pretty good at it. We can walk for long distances too. The world record for the longest walk in 24 hours is 228km. To put that in perspective, Ireland is around 260km coast to coast. Before the 19th century, walking was more or less our only option when on land. That or ride a donkey or horse or be pulled along slowly in a cart. I think it's safe to assume that our ancestors spent much time walking.

Philosopher Fredrich Nietzsche once said, "All truly great thoughts are conceived while walking." And he wasn't the only great mind that placed a high value on walking. Albert Einstein, Charles Darwin, Virginia Woolf, Socrates, Aristotle, and Beethoven all believed in the power of walking. Today science and psychologists concur.

Did you know . . . Barefoot shoes can help you walk more naturally

I've been wearing barefoot shoes for several years, and I love them. Many modern shoe designs constrict your feet and provide unnatural cushions for your feet, which can lead to unnatural movement. Barefoot shoes take some getting used to but will result in stronger feet and ankles and a more natural gait.

Our minds and bodies are not entirely separate entities. Moving your body also gets your mind moving. Anecdotally, I've found that whenever I get stuck on some complex software design question or difficult-to-solve bugs when writing computer code, a short walk will often provide the answer. If I'm feeling bad, a short walk will make me feel a bit better. If I'm feeling good, getting outside will leave me feeling great.

Interestingly, I've also found that conversation tends to flow more smoothly for me when walking with someone, compared to just sitting in a room with them. I'm not sure why.

I just suddenly have a lot to say. So, there is value in both: walking alone and finding companions.

A recent study conducted by Stanford researchers also suggested that creative thinking improves with walking and that indoor and outdoor walking can significantly boost creative inspiration.[4] It seems that the act of walking itself, rather than the environment, is the main factor influencing creativity. The study also revealed that creative thinking continued even after participants stopped walking.

Then there are the health benefits. Walking is great for reducing body fat, lowering blood sugar, reducing the risk of heart disease, supporting your immune system, increasing energy, increasing the strength of your legs, and much more.[5] I think most people have heard about these benefits plenty of times, and all of it is borne out by a plethora of scientific research. A quick search on PubMed for the word "Walking" yields over 12,000 results. But I'm not going to go into that. What's the point? How often has a bunch of scientific research convinced you to do something? I firmly believe that you're better off going and feeling the benefits for yourself. You have agency here. Don't walk because you were told it's good for you. Try it for a couple of weeks and make your own mind up.

4 Wong, M. Stanford Study Finds Walking Improves Creativity. Stanford News. 24 April, 2014.
 https://news.stanford.edu/2014/04/24/walking-vs-sitting-042414/
5 Arthritis Foundation. 12 Benefits of Walking. https://www.arthritis. org/health-wellness/healthy-living/physical-activity/walking/12-benefits-of-walking

This isn't homework; it's an opportunity.

I should also add that I have an additional incentive here that makes going for a walk an easier activity to maintain. I've had days where walking is really painful. My hips and lower back screaming at me with every step. The lower vertebrae of my spine feel like they're made out of paper, and my hips feel like they're going to split in two. On those days, I still go for a walk, though I have to make a conscious effort to brace my stomach and glute muscles as I move; I need as much help from my breath and muscles as I can get. On those days, I really appreciate walking, as in the ability to walk. On those days, a less mobile life flashes before my eyes. A life where I can't walk. And on those days, I work extra hard to make sure that the day that I lose agency, the day where I lose the ability to move and look after myself, never comes. As such, walking has also become a practice of gratitude for what I do have. I've come to truly believe that walking is a privilege and one of life's simple pleasures.

Advisory: It's a good idea to check with your medical practitioner before starting any new exercise regime.

Putting the Strategy into Practice

I'm not sure there is anything you can do in life that has a lower barrier to entry than walking. But, as with everything I talk about here, consistency is key. Going for a walk once every six months won't do much for you. A 10-minute walk every day, on the other hand, could be life-changing. But there is one important detail here. I don't think walking with a purpose is the same as just walking. I'm talking about that walk to school or work, where the focus is on the destination, and the walking is just a necessary evil, where you're in a rush, and every person and road is an obstacle just slowing you down. That sort of walk is different.

The daily walk with real value is where time doesn't matter much. Where there is no destination. Where you're just moving through time and space with no real purpose. Whether alone or with someone else, although ideally, some combination of both.

Did you know . . . You can get more bang for your buck by rucking

Another thing that I think is worth trying is "rucking". Go for a walk but add some weight. Put a few kilos worth of stuff in a bag, throw it on your back, and go walking. The additional weight will cause your heart rate to run much higher. You will be tired and out of breath, which will make you stronger and increase your physical capacity. And then, of course, you will get to my favourite part: taking the bag off your back. Your nervous system will have gotten used to that weight, so when you take it off, you will have a brief moment where you feel like you're floating. Your body will just feel lighter. I love this feeling – the reduced pressure across all of the joints in my body, if even just for a moment.

I recommend incorporating a 10–15 minute walk every day or on as many days as possible. Consistency is key. That's where the benefits are, which seems true of all things worth doing. I also find that walking first thing in the morning is hugely beneficial. Getting some morning sunlight into your eyes and onto your skin is incredibly good for you and really sets your day up in the right way. Walking after a meal is also good and can help digestion. If I could do only one of the six strategies outlined here, walking would be it.

Did you know . . . Being in nature is a mood-booster

During the COVID-19 pandemic, researchers from the UK Centre for Ecology and Hydrology recruited 500 volunteers from the UK who engaged in 10-minute nature-based activities at least five times over eight days. The activities included participating in citizen science projects and "nature-noticing" ("where volunteers spent at least 10 minutes in a natural green space, looking and listening to the world around them, and writing down three positive things they observed"). The participants completed surveys before the project, one week after, and two months later. The findings showed that all volunteers reported higher levels of wellbeing and a stronger connection to nature after participating in the project. Moreover, those engaging in nature-noticing activities were likelier to adopt pro-nature behaviours, such as planting pollinator-friendly plants or creating wildlife shelters. The researchers concluded that active engagement with nature, whether through mindful moments or citizen science, is beneficial for

wellbeing and strengthens the human-nature relationship.[6]

So why not try getting out for a walk today? Even if it's just
10 minutes. Find a podcast you'd like to listen to, an audio-
book, or the latest release from your favourite band and get
out there. But I'd like you to do one thing for me. After your
walk, when you get home, sit down and close your eyes and
really try to notice how you're feeling. Can you feel the blood
pumping through your body? Is your mind clearer? Do you
feel more or less stressed than before the walk? Taking the
time to cultivate this awareness of how walking makes you
feel will help you to be consistent, even on those days you
don't feel like going for a walk.

6 British Science Association. New Research Reveals Wellbeing Benefits
of Connecting with Nature. https://www.britishscienceassociation.org/
news/new-research-reveals-wellbeing-benefits-of-connecting-with-na-
ture

2. EAT

"If we could give every individual the right amount of nourishment and exercise, not too little and not too much, we would have the safest way to health."

Hippocrates

Giving Your Body What It Needs

Thrive by upgrading your plate.

My most important realisation about food was that the old maxim "You are what you eat" is the literal truth. Your food gives your body the energy and raw materials it needs to create new cells and repair old ones. And fruit, fish, meat, dairy, nuts, seeds, and vegetables are the raw materials our bodies have been built with for millennia.

Healthier Choices

Over the past couple of hundred years, we've created all manner of processed foods and refined versions of naturally occurring substances (i.e., grains, oils, and sugars). Over the last fifty years, we've taken this to a whole new level, to the point where our diets are predominantly processed. The reality here is that we just don't know the long-term impact of eating like this, we haven't been doing it that long, but the early indicators are not good. Inflammatory conditions (like psoriasis and arthritis) are rising, as are diabetes type 2, heart disease, and cancer. Research in China has shown that someone born in 1990 would have twice the risk of colon cancer and four times the risk of rectal cancer compared to someone born in 1950.[7]

Making matters more complicated is that food has been big business since the 1960s, and in recent years what we eat has somehow become a controversial and, oddly enough, political topic. I don't want to add fuel to that fire, though, so I won't. I'm just going to talk about some of my experiences and provide some insights into how I learned to eat well and, as a result, feel and perform better than ever before.

Here are some things we know our bodies need:

- **Protein** (meat, fish, dairy, beans, and pulses) to maintain muscle mass, which is important for living a long, healthy, mobile life – especially if you have a condition like arthritis.

- **Fibre** (veggies, fruit, pulses, and whole grains) for smooth digestion and gut health, which has a bunch of knock-on effects on our physical and mental health.

- **Fats**, particularly omega-3 (found in oily fish and some nuts), for the brain, nervous system, and joint health.

- **Vitamins and minerals** (found in all whole foods that are sources of proteins, fibre, and fats) to maintain a healthy body and protect it from disease.

7 Pan Z, Huang J, Huang M, et al. Risk Factors for Early-Onset Colorectal Cancer: A Large-Scale Chinese Cohort Study. Journal of the National Cancer Center, 2023; 3(1): 28-34. ISSN 2667-0054, https://doi.org/10.1016/j.jncc.2023.01.001.

Unsurprisingly we can get all of those things by eating the things that humans have been eating for tens of thousands of years: whole foods – meat, fish, vegetables, fruit, nuts, and seeds. Also, unsurprisingly, cutting out processed foods and focusing my diet on these more natural foods has had a hugely positive impact on me personally. But it didn't happen overnight. I spent years adjusting my diet and learning what did and didn't work for me.

Here's what does work:

~ Lots of vegetables: Fibre, plus the range of vitamins and minerals in fibrous foods, play a leading role in my diet. When I have digestive issues, they almost always come with joint pain. (I will routinely eat an entire head of broccoli daily!)

~ Eggs and fish: These are my primary source of protein; they are light and easily digested.

~ Eating slowly: Digestion starts in the mouth, so chewing every mouthful helps avoid indigestion. It also helps to not eat to the point of feeling bloated.

~ Not eating for a few hours before bed.

~ Nut butter and fruit for satiating snacks: Peanut butter smeared on an apple or some dates tastes amazing and is minimally processed.

And here's what doesn't work:

~ Sugar-laden foods: Sugary pastries and chocolate will almost certainly make me sore. That doesn't mean none . . . but sugary drinks, juices, etc., are out.

~ Greasy foods: Interestingly, I used to suffer a lot from heartburn, but that disappeared once I cut out sausages. I rarely get heartburn now, but if I do, it's usually when I'm eating out, and the food is a bit greasy.
~ Refined grains: Too much bread, especially white bread, tends to make me sore.

It's worth noting that every item on the list that doesn't work for me is a food that you would generally find on a list of "inflammatory foods", so it makes sense that they wouldn't work for me. Certain foods contain substances that promote inflammation, which can worsen the pain, swelling, and stiffness associated with arthritis. Remember, psoriatic arthritis (and rheumatoid arthritis, along with many other chronic conditions) result from chronic inflammation. My experience in this case lines up with the research.

And again, this is my experience. This is not a prescription for you. The message I really want to get across is to not un-derestimate the impact of what you're eating on how you feel. Especially if you have arthritis or some other inflammatory condition. Generally speaking, when you eat clean, unpro-cessed foods, you will feel better and healthier. You may also be less likely to depend on prescription drugs and painkillers (Big Pharma) to live your life. To me, that is hugely import-ant. I want agency and freedom. So, in the words of Hippo-crates: "Let thy food be thy medicine and thy medicine be thy food."

Did you know . . . Keeping a food journal can be eye-opening

Food journals are a simple yet powerful tool that can help transform your relationship with food. The information you track can be as simple or as detailed as you like, and you don't need to do it forever, but it's a useful exercise to do from time to time to help calibrate your understanding of what you're putting in your body. Here are just a few of the benefits of keeping a food journal:

Heightened Awareness and Mindful Eating: Keeping a food journal cultivates an awareness of your eating habits. By recording what you consume throughout the day, you'll become more conscious of your choices. And this will help you see patterns, triggers, and habits that may negatively impact your day-to-day life. As you develop a deeper understanding of your relationship with food, you can make better-informed decisions about any changes you'd like to make and track your progress against any goals you might have.

Accountability and Weight Management: A food journal is an honest accountability partner. By documenting meals and snacks, you'll clearly understand your daily nutritional intake. This self-reflection helps identify areas where you may be falling short or overindulging.

Identification of Allergies and Sensitivities: A food journal can help us identify potential food allergies or sensitivities. By recording your meals and any associated symptoms, such as bloating, pain, fatigue, or digestive distress, you can recognise patterns and correlations.

Personalised Nutrition Insights: A food journal can help you understand what foods leave you feeling good and full of energy, and what foods leave you feeling tired, bloated and irritable.

Putting the Strategy into Practice

In the following section, I've outlined some thoughts and insights from my journey from industrial food machine foods to local fresh whole foods. If you are a fussy eater or struggle with food, as I did, this might be useful. Again, there is no judgement here. You need to decide what matters to you. The important takeaway is that food is powerful in many ways, so it's worth thinking about.

I was a fussy eater growing up. As with most picky eaters, this means my diet was seriously lacking in nutrients and consisted largely of processed food. My plate was generally beige and bland. Chicken and potatoes. Bread and cheese. Sausages and chips (fries). Chicken in a bread roll.

Over the past decade or so, that has shifted dramatically in the complete opposite direction. I will happily eat pretty much any fruit or vegetable put in front of me. My diet is more diverse, flavourful, and nutrient-dense than ever, though I didn't make it easy on myself or my girlfriend, whose encouragement often led to greater resistance from me. But it's worth mentioning that I didn't plan any of this; it just happened over time. Though looking back on it now, I can identify a few key things that changed my mindset when it came to food. But first, here are a few observations about my own struggle to adopt a healthier diet and lifestyle:

- **It's all in your head:** The hardest barrier to overcome is often the mental one. I would look at some foods and decide I didn't like them. I knew that the food wouldn't kill me, but I refused to even try it. It was a mental barrier that I had built up over decades. This is a psychological phenomenon, so don't trivialise it by thinking, "Oh, I'm just picky." It's not easy to get over, so don't expect it to be.

- **It's not just taste, it's texture:** Often, my issue with certain foods was not how they tasted but how they felt in my mouth.

- **It's you vs the global food industry:** Don't be too hard on yourself if you struggle to make healthy changes to your diet; it's an uphill battle. The food industry uses various psychological tricks to get you to buy processed, sugar, and fat-laden foods. Coupled with the modern busy and stressful lives many of us lead, it's harder than ever to eat healthily, despite the bombardment of "healthy" food labels in the supermarket.

So here is some practical advice on how to make healthy changes to your diet.

Learn About Food and Cooking

The one thing I found to be the most effective tool in the fight against an unhealthy lifestyle was learning more about food and nutrition. This happened when I moved out of my parents' house and had to start cooking for myself. Thankfully I didn't just resign myself to frozen dinners and fast food takeouts; I started to prepare food myself. I quickly got bored and wanted to try new dishes, so I had to learn more about food. What I quickly discovered is that I really enjoy cooking. While I find it somewhat cathartic, I appreciate that this won't be the case for everyone. If you really can't stand cooking, I would suggest finding four or five quick and easy main dishes and cycling through them week to week. Over time you will get confident enough to start making tweaks and experimenting with new things. These were my go-to dishes for a long time:

- **Stir fry**: It doesn't get much easier than this. Throw some vegetables and a bit of protein (fish, meat, or tofu) in a pan, and add soy sauce and rice or noodles. You can add healthy fats with a sprinkle of toasted seeds.

- **Wholegrain pasta with mixed vegetables**: Once you can make a tasty sauce, you can use it for various dishes. Avoid store-bought sauces as they are often filled with sugar. To make a tasty traditional pasta sauce, you only need a small onion, a jar of passata, and a stock cube. Finely chop the onion and gently fry until translucent. Add the passata and a stock cube and allow to heat through gently. That's it. If you're adding meat, add to the onion and cook it before adding the passata. Or you might want to spice it up by adding herbs and garlic or some finely chopped carrot and celery to the onions as they're cooking.

- **Curries, chillis, and stews** (pot cooking in general): Get yourself a decent Dutch oven. Pot cooking is super easy and can produce amazing results. A good Dutch oven is a purchase that will last you for life, so don't be afraid to spend the money to get a good one.

- **Soup**: You can't beat soup during the winter. Embarrassingly, I didn't start eating soup until my mid-twenties. You can make your own healthy soup by throwing a bunch of veg in boiling water with a stock cube, simmering until it is cooked, and then blending it.

Once I started cooking more, I also started to pay attention to the ingredients in store-bought processed foods. I began to wonder why all that extra crap was in there and why I never needed to add things like "silicon dioxide" (anti-caking) or "dextrose" (sugar) to my own dishes.

Did you know . . . That sugar goes by more than 50 names

Sugar, in its various forms, is an omnipresent ingredient in our modern diet. While many of us strive to limit our sugar intake, we often encounter a challenging hurdle: the many names used to disguise its presence. Understanding the various aliases that food manufacturers use for sugar can help us make more informed choices.

Here are just a few of the many names you might see on food labels that all basically mean one thing – added sugar:

- Sucrose
- High fructose corn syrup
- Dextrin
- Dextrose
- Glucose
- Maltodextrin
- Maltose
- Lactose

Excess sugar consumption can lead to chronic low-grade inflammation and corresponding health concerns. If you are living with an autoimmune condition, like psoriatic or rheumatoid arthritis, then it is important to be aware of the impact of eating sugar on your body.

You should also be aware that many foods labelled "low fat" or "low calorie" often have a lot of added sugar, despite the packaging that may lead you to believe the food is healthier.

Introduce New Healthy Foods Gradually

Don't take on too much at once; this is a great way to set yourself up for failure. Give yourself reasonable short-term goals along with loftier long-term ones. This idea is effective and can be applied to any goal you want to achieve, but it requires consistency and persistence.

Nothing worthwhile has ever happened overnight, so recognise that you need to be in this for the long term.

Instead of sitting down one Sunday night and saying to yourself, *"This week, I'm going to eat only healthy foods,"* aim to introduce one new healthy food to your diet each week. One week you might try to make sure you eat a piece of fruit every day. Maybe the next week you try to drink more water and fewer sugary drinks. Next, you can try at least one new vegetable during the week. Focus on what you are adding rather than what you are restricting.

If you have a bad day full of junk food, so be it. Just try to eat a little healthier the next. The worst thing you can do is set unrealistic goals and beat yourself up for failing. That's more likely to make you ashamed and return to bad habits. Instead, celebrate your wins.

If you're a complete veggie phobe like I was, some vegetables are much easier to start with than others.

- **Bell peppers (also known as capsicum):** These are nice and sweet, with a great crunch if you don't overcook them. The sweetness and crunch mean they will be familiar in flavour and texture, making them a great vegetable to include in your salads, stir-fries, and one-pot dinners.

- **Carrots:** Steamed or stir-fried carrots don't have an overpowering flavour, are a little sweet, and have a nice crunch if not overcooked. Like peppers, they are a great vegetable and go with everything.

- **Spinach:** This is easily the best green leafy vegetable to start with. It has a mild flavour, goes with any-thing, and is nutrient dense.

- **Broccoli:** If you cut up broccoli florets and stir fry them, they are very inoffensive to your taste buds. They are generally regarded as a "superfood" because they are nutrient-dense. Broccoli is part of the cruciferous family of vegetables, which some research suggests has anti-cancer properties. It's hard to think of a reason not to start eating broccoli.

These were my staple vegetables for a long time and are a solid foundation to build on. Once you are comfortable with spinach, it is easy to branch out to all manner of salad leaves and other dark green leafy veg. Once comfortable with carrots, you can try other root vegetables like beetroot or parsnips.

It takes time for your palette to change, so be patient and introduce vegetables slowly. Doing something, regardless of how small it is, is infinitely better than doing nothing, so there's nothing wrong with slow and steady as long as you are consistent. Cut out junk and slowly introduce fruit and vegetables, and your tastes will change in a few weeks, as will your body and health.

Texture Takes Time

Most vegetables don't actually have a strong taste. We are much more sensitive to sweet-tasting fruits or the spices we add to our cooking. Once I realised this, I was more open to trying new things. Texture, however, was a different story, and I still struggle with it.

Take bell peppers, for example. I love them raw, cooked in a sauce, or stir-fried. If you roast them, however, they lose their appeal entirely. Roasting makes them more flavourful and sweeter – they taste amazing – but it also changes their texture. It makes them soft and a little slimy to me. This is where my problem lies. The same goes for aubergine (eggplant) and even tomatoes. I love the taste of tomatoes but have to cut away the centre portion.

Remember that there are many different ways to prepare vegetables, so even if you think you don't like any given vegetable, you can try preparing it differently. I found that stir-frying generally yielded a texture I liked; this may or may not be the same for you.

Just remember that texture and taste are two different things. This battle is fought on two fronts, and for me, the texture is the tougher mental battle. I'm still working on texture and have become more open to roasted peppers, which I hope will be a gateway to other vegetables and preparation methods that produce similar textures.

It's also worth remembering that the highly palatable processed foods we're surrounded by are created by food scientists and are literally designed to feel good in your mouth. It's hard to compete with that. But you can. Real food can and will feel better to you over time.

Bring Willpower to the Supermarket, Forget It at Home

It is easier to say no once in the supermarket than ten times at home. If you only have healthy food in your house, you must eat healthy. On the other hand, if your house is full of junk food, you must constantly fight the urge to eat it. If, for example, you buy a pack of ten of your favourite chocolate bar because they were on special offer, it means you have to try and resist that urge ten times at home. However, in the supermarket, you only have to resist that urge once. When you're at home, you might regret not buying them, but if you're trying to stay away from that sort of thing, then you'd regret eating them a lot more.

Don't Shop on an Empty Stomach

I think this is just good advice in general. If you are starving while cruising the supermarket aisles, you will be more tempted to buy the things you are trying to avoid. Special offers for oven pizzas or sweet snacks will be harder to resist if your stomach and brain are screaming at you to buy them.

Hunger is the Best Sauce

Avoid snacking so that you are good and hungry for your main meals. This is more important in the early days. If you are properly hungry, you will eat anything – even those vegetables you thought you hated. This can be hugely beneficial, provided everything you eat is nutritious and healthy. I'm not suggesting that you starve yourself, but if you eat three decent square meals a day and include some moderate activity in your daily routine, then you will be less picky with your food. The key is to be hungry and limit your options.

Something else I often recommend to people is trying a vegetarian diet for a month. Not for any sort of ideological reason but purely for the sake of limiting your options. If you go to a restaurant and they only have one vegetarian option, then you have to try it. This can effectively broaden your horizons as you are forced to adapt and change how you eat.

Food and Fitness Go Hand in Hand

We'll talk about exercise in more depth in the next section, but it's worth mentioning because fitness and nutrition are inseparable in many ways. When you start to enjoy exercise and give yourself some fitness goals, whether it's to run a marathon or deadlift 200kg, you quickly realise that you need to get your nutrition in order if you want to succeed. Fitness goals create nutrition goals. Without proper nutrition, you cannot get your body to perform at its best.

I recommend doing any exercise so that when those cravings for unhealthy food appear, you have a counterbalance. You have a reason not to succumb. That ice cream or piece of chocolate will wipe out anything you may have gained from today's 5km run. You will be motivated by your own actions – and that is sustainable.

Supplements

Do you need to supplement your diet?

The answer is that it depends.

For performance (i.e., sport & fitness)? No, probably not. Many people will try to sell supplements to you, but you probably don't need them. Not now, anyway. When approaching an elite level of athleticism, you'd probably want to take some advice on the best supplements to add to your diet, but before then, probably not.

For health? Yes, probably. If you do not eat meat or animal products, it would probably be a good idea to supplement protein, and B12 supplementation will be essential. In fact, most people could do with supplementing B12 and vitamin D. If you have any joint issues, it would be a good idea to take some krill or cod liver oil tablets daily.

Action List

The best way to get all the nutrients you need is to eat a well-balanced diet; it really is that simple.

If I were to give you an action list, it would look like this:

~ Prepare and cook your own food, this is an invaluable life skill, and you'll eat better and for less money.
~ Eat fruit and veg. Aim for the rainbow – plenty of different colours!
~ Don't drink your calories in fizzy drinks and/or alcohol.
~ Limit refined sugar as much as possible.

When it comes to planning your meals, try to stick to the following rough guideline for portion size:

~ One palm-sized portion of protein (eggs, chicken, tofu, lentils, etc.)
~ One fist-size portion of vegetables (broccoli, peas, carrots, green beans, tomatoes, leafy greens, salad etc.).
~ Cupped hand-size portion of starchy carbs (beans, potatoes, rice, sweet potato, quinoa, whole meal bread, etc.)
~ One thumb size portion of fat (avocado, oils, salad dressing, nuts).

That's it for food. Unfortunately, I can't do all of this for you; you need to go exploring and learn for yourself. Hopefully, through simple dietary changes, you can find more well-being and fewer, or less severe, flare-ups.

"Eat food. Not too much. Mostly plants."

~ Michael Pollan

3. Move

"Flexibility is the key to stability."

John Wooden

Where the Mind Meets the Body

Stretch into more mobility

"I am not flexible." I used to tell myself this all the time. In hindsight, it's a pretty silly statement. Flexibility isn't a thing you just have. Sure, some people are naturally more flexible than others, but being flexible is not an innate trait. I have blue eyes and dark hair. I also have light skin that damages easily in the sun. Those things are innate truths. Flexibility, on the other hand, is different. My thinking I was inflexible is akin to thinking, "I can't play the trumpet." It's true. I can't play the trumpet. But I've also never tried and have never had a desire to. I can, however, play the guitar. Not very well, but I wanted to learn, so I did. It took lots of practice over many years, and I could be a lot better, but I was inconsistent and never sought out a teacher. I've just had fun with it. The point I'm making here is that it's important to keep an open mind about what you can and can't do. And the exact same logic can and should be applied to flexibility.

Open-minded Thinking

For the longest time, I couldn't touch my toes. I could just about manage to touch my shins. These days, however, I can place my hands flat on the floor while keeping my legs completely locked out. It just took time and consistent effort. Though it wasn't that much effort. I just started stretching a little in the evenings before bed. I did it while watching TV, so nothing really changed. I was sitting on the floor doing some stretches instead of sitting on the couch doing nothing. Well, probably not nothing, perhaps flicking through my phone while whatever was on TV struggled to maintain my full attention.

Just 10 minutes before bed, that was basically it. But I was consistent. Then I'd throw in a few stretches throughout the day too. At work, when I went to the toilet, I'd stand in the cubicle and stretch for a minute or two. If I was making some tea, I'd stretch while waiting for the kettle to boil. It just became a habit, and within a few months, I got to my toes!

But something else happened around that time. All I really wanted was to touch my toes, but what I got was a general overall improvement in how I moved. So, I looked for other areas where I had limitations. My shoulders were particularly bad, and my hips too. Years of sitting, hunched over, and mashing keys on a keyboard tend to have this effect. I went to work on those body parts too, but I learned quickly that stretching everything all the time is not necessarily a great idea.

There's flexibility, and there's mobility; they're different and both important.

Flexibility vs Mobility

Flexibility involves getting your joints into their end range of motion. This is where you can no longer move any deeper into the stretch. You can, however, increase this end range by physically pulling yourself into it. For example, imagine you put your foot up on a table with your leg straight and then have a friend lift your leg and place a number of books under it until they can no longer lift your leg any higher.

You might be tempted to say, "Look how high I can lift my leg!" But you didn't lift your leg that high, not really. If you remove the books and the table, your leg will likely come crashing down. You were flexible enough to get your leg up there with a whole lot of support but not mobile enough to keep it there when the support is removed.

Mobility is all about exercising control at your end range of motion. And it is difficult. Improving mobility is hard work. Cramps and frustration await as your muscles just flat-out re-fuse to do what you're trying to tell them to do. It's really easy to try this out for yourself. Stand up and take your right foot in your right hand so that you can pull your foot toward your ass. This should be pretty doable for most people. The goal is to have it so that the back of your leg above the knee is touch-ing the back of your leg below the knee. In this position, you should feel a stretch in front of that same leg. Now, slowly let go with your right hand, but try to keep your right leg in the same position. To do this, you will have to really fire up the muscles in the back of your leg (your hamstring muscles).

What happened? Your foot almost certainly fell away from your ass as soon as you let go. This is because you are flexible enough to put your leg in that position but not mobile enough to keep it there on its own. If you have good muscle control and can really engage your hamstring muscles, this will probably cause a cramp.

Mobility work appeals to me because controlling my muscles helps manage the pain in my joints. What's interesting about this work is that you're actually training your brain. You are improving the connections between your brain and your muscles. Those connections are part of your central nervous system, which fires electrical signals around your body. If you lack control over your muscles, it means that the signals that your brain is sending them are weak.

I believe mobility and flexibility training provides the perfect opportunity to set some fitness goals. When it comes to health and fitness, it's easy to fall into the trap of thinking that the only metric to measure progress is the scales. How much we weigh, or what our body fat percentage is. I don't like the scales; it's misleading. I much prefer movement and strength-related goals. Can I walk 10km without stopping? Can I touch my toes? Can I do 10 pull-ups?

Having movement and strength-related goals lets us focus on what we're gaining, not losing.

With flexibility and mobility, the scale is less relevant. You don't do this to lose weight or build muscle. You do it to feel and move better. Excess weight might get in the way, but that is a separate discussion, and you can still work on mobility and flexibility despite that.

Here are some goals that you can think about working towards, and you can make a lot of progress with just a small daily investment:

~ Touch your toes.
~ Put on your socks in the morning while standing without using any support.
~ Stand up from a seated position without using your arms.
~ Get out of bed without using your arms.
~ Get down on the floor and back up again, only using one arm.
~ Get down on the floor and back up again without using your arms.
~ Sit in a deep squat position for a minute or more.

The Mind-Body Connection

Most of the time, we don't think about our nervous system. It just works. If I tell you to lift your arm, you don't have to put any thought into which muscles your brain is going to recruit to actually lift your arm. If you did, you wouldn't really have the time to think about or indeed do anything else with your life. But it's important to know that your body can and will learn bad movement patterns too. In fact, it's a lot easier to train your body to move poorly than to train it to move well. This often happens when people get injured.

For example, if you injure your foot, you may start walking in a way that takes the weight off it. Do that for long enough, and it will become "the way you walk". Over months and years, this unnatural movement pattern can harm your joints and lead to further injury. Something as simple as trying to carry all your shopping in from the car in one trip could cause you to hurt your hip. Or maybe you're moving some furniture to get the vacuum cleaner behind it and throw it out your back. The longer you live with these bad movement patterns, the harder, and possibly more painful, it gets to change them.

If, like me, you have arthritis, it is vital that you control how you move. That you try to program your body in a way that allows it to move well. If you don't have arthritis, then doing this is still a good idea. Think of it as insurance. You will be more resilient and less likely to injure yourself. I'm going to throw out a terrifying fact here to try and emphasise this point: falls are the leading cause of injury-related deaths among persons aged ≥65 years, and the age-adjusted rate of deaths from falls is increasing. In 2016, a total of 29,668 U.S. residents aged ≥65 years died as a result of a fall.[8]

Did you know . . . How to avoid falls

Falls can lead to serious injuries and significantly impact your quality of life. By incorporating exercises that improve balance, stability, and coordination, you can enhance your ability to maintain equilibrium and react appropriately to potential fall hazards. Balance

8 Burns E, Kakara R. Deaths from Falls Among Persons Aged ≥65 Years — United States, 2007–2016. MMWR Morb Mortal Wkly Rep 2018; 67:509–514. DOI: http://dx.doi.org/10.15585/mmwr.mm6718a1

training exercises, such as standing on one leg, walking heel-to-toe, or practising yoga, help strengthen the muscles that maintain balance and promote better overall stability. By regularly engaging in such exercises, you can improve your body awareness and physical control and so reduce the risk of falls.

Mobility exercises enhance strength, flexibility, and range of motion, allowing you to move more confidently and efficiently. Strengthening the lower body muscles, such as the quadriceps and hamstrings, through exercises like squats and lunges can improve walking stability and prevent missteps that may lead to falls. Flexibility exercises, including stretching the hip, knee, and ankle joints, promote greater freedom of movement and reduce stiffness that can impede mobility. By regularly engaging in balance and mobility training, you can enhance your physical capacity, increase your self-confidence, and significantly reduce the risk of falls, ultimately improving your overall safety and well-being.

Putting the Strategy into Practice

As mentioned earlier in the book, I have practised yoga and Pilates to improve my flexibility and mobility. Both practices also help you to build some strength and will teach you how to effectively incorporate breathing into your movements.

As with everything else, consistency is key to improving your flexibility and mobility. A short pre-bed or early morning routine works. Just 10 minutes a day will add up quickly. However, I wouldn't recommend just jumping in as I would with walking or trying different foods. I think it's important to get some guidance here. This could be in the form of two or three yoga classes or a month of Pilates with an instructor, or working with a mobility coach for a while. Whichever you choose, it will be important to get direct feedback and guidance about how you are moving. Learn how to move properly before starting any longer-term routine. Remember, practice doesn't make perfect; it makes permanent. Perfect practice makes perfect.

It's also worth remembering that this is an investment in yourself, which can yield massive returns. Once you've learned a bit from someone who knows what they are doing, you can start exploring independently. And once you've acquired that ability, it's yours. Forever. No one can take that away from you.

But you can't just attend a few classes and follow along absentmindedly. You have to think about what you're doing. Really think about it. Ask questions. Take notes on what is going on in your body. Is one joint, in particular, giving you trouble? Is one side weaker than the other? Why? Make the absolute most of it. Figure out your weak points and ask your instructor how to tackle them. Ask them to give you a nightly routine to improve. Get your money's worth!

Once you've done that, you'll be ready to turn to the many resources available online to grow your knowledge. You will be doing this having already gained enough knowledge to know what to look for. This is vital as you will need to be able to filter through the crap because there is a lot of crap out there.

Did you know . . . Your ego is best left at the door

The internet, in particular, is a very misleading place. Not least of all, there are a lot of dedicated people out there that are so good at this flexibility stuff that they make it look really easy. We watch them and conclude that it must be easy because it looks easy. It's not. Focus on the fundamentals and avoid the flashy stuff. And it's not just that people are making it look easy. There are also many people trying to sell you shortcuts and hacks. There are none. I've looked. They don't exist. Your mind is much easier to fool than your body. You need to give your body the time it needs, and that's the end of it, really.

When building an exercise routine, most of us need to work on our shoulders, back, and hips. We sit a lot with our shoulders rounded forward. This is a recipe for tight hips, poor posture, and back pain. Spend time opening your hips, extending your back, and pulling your shoulders back and down. Yoga and Pilates naturally address all of these things, but you can create specific routines that target each area and only take 10 minutes. Ideally, you should spend as long as you can, but 10 minutes every day is good. That will get you a long, long way. Remember, we're not trying to join Cirque du Soleil here, you don't need to spend all day doing this, but you need to do something, especially if you're battling arthritis.

4. Lift

"If you think lifting is dangerous, try being weak. Being weak is dangerous."

~ Bret Contreras

Strength Is Everything

Push your body and mind

I'm going to start with an uncomfortable truth . . . Unless you do or have done some sort of resistance training (i.e., calisthenics or lifting weights), you have no idea how physically weak you are or how strong you can be. This section is all about getting stronger. That's what resistance training, for me at least, is all about. Sure, you can do this stuff to build muscle, lose weight, get a beach body, or whatever body you want looking back at you in the mirror, but for me, those are just pleasant side effects. Strength is everything, especially if you have arthritis. You need to take the load off your joints and put it on your muscles. Get strong, and everything else – literally everything else – will be easier. For years, I've been trying to think of just one downside to being physically stronger and have yet to come up with anything. If you can think of some-thing, please let me know.

Stressbusting

At this point, resistance training has become meditative for me. Oddly enough, it is something I do to relax. I always feel better after weight training. Mentally and physically. Whatever stress exists in my life just seems to evaporate. This shouldn't really be a surprise if you think about it. When you push your body hard, your mind is happy enough to take a back seat. For example, I'm never too worried about the stresses of work while holding a 32kg kettlebell over my head, as 100 per cent of my focus is on that thing in my hand that, if I dropped on my foot, would crush every single bone inside of it (or potentially kill me if I dropped it on my head!). When lifting, you usually live in the present moment, and it's not too often that you get to do that.

Did you know ... Mindfulness can happen anywhere

Mindfulness is a practice that involves intentionally bringing your attention to the present moment with an attitude of openness and non-judgment. While it is often associated with meditation, mindfulness can be practised in various ways to suit different preferences and lifestyles. You can cultivate mindfulness through walking, eating, or everyday tasks like washing dishes or brushing your teeth. The key is to bring awareness and focused attention to the present experience, observing thoughts, sensations, and emotions without getting caught up in them. By practising mindfulness in different ways, you can find a method that resonates with you and integrate it into your day-to-day life.

Engaging in regular mindfulness practice offers numerous benefits for both mental and physical health. Research has shown that mindfulness can reduce stress, anxiety, and depression by promoting a greater sense of calm and relaxation. It can help you develop resilience and respond to challenging situations with clarity and composure. Mindfulness practice can also improve cognitive functions such as attention, memory, and decision-making. By training your mind to stay present and focused, you can enhance your productivity and overall cognitive performance. Mindfulness has also been found to positively affect physical health, such as reducing blood pressure, boosting immune function, and promoting better sleep.[9]

The beauty of mindfulness lies in its accessibility and adaptability. It can be practised by anyone, regardless of age or background, and can be incorporated into various aspects of life. Whether dedicating a few minutes each day to formal meditation, taking mindful breaks during the workday, or infusing mindfulness into routine activities, the practice offers an opportunity to cultivate a deeper connection with yourself and the present moment. By fostering mindfulness, you can experience improved well-being, reduced stress levels, enhanced cognitive abilities, and a greater sense of harmony.

Beware the Fitness Industry

Before I go any further, however, I want to take a moment to talk about the fitness industry. Put simply, it has problems. The industry has many charlatans pushing information that

9 Dorwart L. The Health Benefits of Mindfulness. Health.com. 26. April 2023. https://www.health.com/benefits-of-mindfulness-7480142

is, at best misleading, at worst dangerous. Everywhere you turn, you will find people telling you that the supplement they are more than happy to sell to you is all you need to go from scrawny weakling to muscle-bound action movie star. More often than not, these so-called fitness gurus use steroids, lie about it, and then try to sell you their product, whatever it is, claiming that it is all you need to get a body like theirs. Generally speaking, you would do well to avoid most Instagram fitness influencers. Anyone that tells you that their product will help you lose 20kg of fat in two weeks or gain 10kg of muscle in 30 days is straight-up lying to you.

You will also find people using words like "shred" or "beast mode", or videos of people exhausting themselves to the point where they are a sweaty mess, laid out on the floor. Then they will offer banal motivational quotes that might make you feel good for a minute or two but don't achieve anything. The grim reality is that motivation isn't worth all that much. It's fleeting. But it's sexy and easy, so a whole mini-industry has grown around it. It's easy to sit around reading motivational quotes and feeling good, all the while you're not actually doing anything. These people will tell you that their fitness level is achievable by using their supplements and following their program. But it's not. They look and perform the way they do because it is their job. They can, and do, spend all day working on themselves, managing a perfect fitness routine because that's what they do. That's what they are selling you. It's aspirational. We want to be like them. But if you have a job and kids and various other life pressures, then it's just not realistic.

Okay, rant over. I just get really frustrated with the amount of confusion and misinformation spread by an industry that, at its core, is meant to help people. And I'd like to present a different view of fitness and strength training to you.

Day-to-Day Strength

My recommendation is to lift weights and work on your fitness because you love yourself, not because you hate your body. It's not a punishment for eating chocolate. It's a way to help your mind and body function better. A way to make it easier for you to perform day-to-day tasks. Tasks as simple as standing out of a chair or opening a jar, or as big as a DIY project that requires a sledgehammer, chopping wood or digging up your garden. I call it "day-to-day strength", and it's very useful to have. And not only that, but you will also improve your movement, your balance, your mental strength, the function of your organs, your metabolism and much more.

Think of it like brushing your teeth. It's not a punishment at the end of the day for all of the eating you did. You do it because it's a damn good idea to maintain healthy teeth. Unfortunately, building strength is a bit more involved than maintaining healthy teeth. With teeth, you can brush a few times a day and hit the dentist twice a year, and you should be good to go.

Strength and fitness training requires
a bit more effort,
especially if you live with arthritis,
but it's worth it.

Before considering how to start implementing this, I want to talk about strength and hypertrophy (building muscle). As

I mentioned earlier in the book, big muscles and strong muscles are not exactly the same thing. You can be strong without giant muscles like those shiny, bronzed bodybuilders at bodybuilding contests. In fact, "bodybuilding" and "strength training" are two different types of training. Neither one is better than the other. They are just different. The end goals are different. Some people want to build a certain physique. Others want to be strong and don't care what they look like. Practically speaking, it will be easier and more useful for the average person to get strong. And if you have arthritis, strength training will help you achieve more well-being, despite the condition.

With bodybuilding, you are trying to force your muscles to get bigger. High volume is the name of the game. This means lots of sets with lots of reps (we'll cover sets and reps later if this terminology means nothing to you). You will often find bodybuilders trying to completely exhaust their muscles. They will also usually incorporate a lot of "isolation" exercises. This is where you do some movement that targets a very specific muscle. For example, a dumbbell curl is an exercise that targets the biceps, which is probably the most famous muscle group. Bodybuilders not only need to spend a lot of time in the gym, but they also need to be really disciplined when it comes to food. They tend to eat a lot of protein and very little in the way of carbohydrates. This helps them reduce the amount of fat they are carrying on their body. They will also go through cycles where they "bulk" (eat a LOT) and then "cut" (eat very little). If you're thinking, *This sounds like a full-time job!* then you're right. It is. Building lots of muscle is hard and takes a lot of time (and usually some anabolic steroids).

When it comes to strength training, you are training your body's neuromuscular system rather than focusing on increasing muscle size. Strength is a skill, and you train a bit differently to increase your skill level. That's not to say bodybuilders are not strong. They are, very much so. But absolute strength is not necessarily their goal.

I'm bringing this up because a lot of the training you see in popular culture comes from bodybuilding. Body composition goals are generally used to sell fitness programs and products. And it makes sense. Lots of people want abs and a big ass. Strength isn't sexy. Watching someone lift something heavy is hard to appreciate unless you've done it yourself and understand the effort involved. But don't worry about all of that stuff for now. Just know that you don't need to hammer your body in the gym day after day to get stronger. In fact, with the right strength training routine, you might walk away from the gym thinking, *"I don't even feel like I really worked out today."*

The message I want to get across here is this: You can get strong, stronger than you can even know right now. And, importantly, you can go a long way with a minimal but consistent time investment, so that's what we will focus on here. But first, a quick side note.

Fat Loss and General Advice

As I've already said, my primary motivation is strength and mobility. However, I appreciate that for many people, the initial motivation for working out may stem from a desire to reduce their body fat or change their body composition. It's also important to keep your body weight in check if you're living with arthritis, as additional weight will increase strain on your joints and impact your ability to stay mobile, so I want to speak to that for a minute.

Cardio (running, cycling, high-intensity workouts, etc.) is often sold as the key to fat loss. The idea is to throw your body around for 30 minutes to an hour to burn off those calories and lose fat. By the end, you are a sweaty mess and can almost feel the fat burning.

This does work, but it is not necessarily the best approach. If you jumped on a rowing machine, you'd have to row pretty hard for 10–15 minutes just to burn off the calories from a banana. A Frappucino from Starbucks could take over an hour of rowing to offset the calories (depending on your toppings).

My point is this: doing cardio to burn off calories is a lot of hard work, and it's not actually all that effective. I'm only talking about fat loss here. There are, of course, other benefits to doing cardio, but if you're trying to lose fat, there are better approaches and strength training is one of them.

To illustrate how this works, I'd like to use an analogy. Imagine you have a car. That car has a full fuel tank or a fully charged battery. Now, imagine that you want to use up all of that fuel and that I have given you two options:

1. You drive the car around really fast for 30 minutes every second day, then turn the engine off when you get home.
2. You drive the car around more slowly for 30 minutes every second day, then leave the engine running when you get home.

Which option are you going to take? If the goal is to use fuel, I would lean toward the second option.

The second option is strength training. As you build strength and consequentially build muscle, you are changing your body's metabolism. Bodies with more muscle require more calories to operate, so it's like leaving your engine running. And I'm not talking about world-champion bodybuilder levels of muscle here; just a small increase in muscle mass will change how many calories your body needs each day. This is called your Basal Metabolic Rate and refers to how many calories your body uses while sitting there doing nothing. So, for example, if you need 2,000 calories per day to maintain your current body weight and energy expenditure and you add some muscle to your body, your caloric needs may increase to something like 2,100 calories per day. If you don't increase your calorie intake, you will be in "calorie deficit", meaning you consume fewer calories than your body needs to maintain its current state. You need to be in a deficit to lose body fat. Going by this example, you could lose body fat without changing your diet because your additional muscle mass is consuming more calories. This is oversimplified; there are, of course, a lot of different factors at play. I just wanted to highlight some ways that muscle can impact how your body works.

So, in short: if you don't really care about strength and just want to lose body fat, strength training may still be your best option. Though it is important to remember that when it comes to fat loss, diet is still where your focus needs to be. It's very difficult to outwork excessive calorie consumption.

I have a couple more general notes about strength training before we put the strategy into practice, and at this point, I will generalise heavily. This may or may not apply to you as a man or woman, but this is common advice you might find helpful.

For Men

Check your ego. Men tend to lift too heavy and do so with poor movement. No one cares how much you can lift, go slowly and do it properly. Lift with good form, and you will get stronger and save a lot of injury pain.

For Women

Don't worry about getting big and bulky; it won't happen unless you want it to and work hard at it. Building muscle is very difficult, and no one has ever built a big and bulky body-builder physique accidentally. This is especially true for women, who tend to have a harder time building muscle anyway.

Putting the Strategy into Practice

Let me start with a story. Around 2,500 years ago, there was a man called Milo. He was from southern Italy and has become a legend. Milo was a six-time Olympic champion renowned for his feats of strength. One day, as a young man, a calf was born near his house. Milo decided to pick this calf up onto his shoulders and go walking with it. He then did this every day for four years. Each day the calf would get bigger, weigh a little more, and he would pick it up and put it on his shoulders. In response to the increased weight of the calf, Milo's body had to adapt. It had to get stronger to accommodate the growing calf. After four years, his strength had increased enough to carry a full-sized bull.

The legend of Milo of Croton, though unrealistic, is a lesson in something called "progressive overload", and it is the foundation of strength training. In essence, you need to put your body under some physical stress, let it adapt to that stress, and then increase it. So how do you do that without carrying a calf everywhere?

First, let's go through some terminology. Entering the world of strength training can be daunting, so let's be clear about how we talk about training so that it's not confusing or overwhelming.

Sets and Reps

Consider the push-up. I think everyone knows what a push-up looks like (though many people execute them pretty poorly). If you do a single push-up, that would be considered "1 rep" (short for repetition). If you do 10 push-ups, then you've done 10 reps.

Then you can do multiple sets of reps. So, for example, if I do ten push-ups and then rest for 1–2 minutes and then do another ten, I will have just done two sets of ten. Personal trainers will often structure their training programs like this. They might say something like "Push-ups – 3 x 10". That is telling you to do three sets of ten reps. Or, more simply: do ten push-ups, rest a bit, do ten more, rest a bit, do ten more.

Resting

You might also be given a defined "resting period." Your rest period is the time between sets. This can greatly impact, among other things, how hard something is. For example, if you do two sets of 10 push-ups with 60 seconds of rest between sets, you can do 10 push-ups, rest for a whole minute, and then do 10 more. However, if this rest period is only 10 seconds, your second set of push-ups will be much harder because your body hasn't had much time to recover. After you exert some effort, your muscles need some time to relax before they return to full strength. And not just your muscles. When lifting heavy weights, your nervous system can need 15 or more minutes to recover!

All your strength training will revolve around manipulating the number of reps and sets you are doing, the weight you are lifting, and how much rest you are getting. I won't go into specifics here as to why this is the case, but decades of strength training experience have informed trainers how to best approach lifting weights for optimal return on investment. If you are following a good program, then this wisdom will be taken into account.

Ok, now that we have the terminology sorted, let's get back to the idea of "progressive overload" and why the story of Milo and his calf was relevant to strength training. Let's once again consider the humble push-up. If you can do 3 push-ups and want to get to 10, how might you do that?

Well, one good way to go about it would be to do three sets of 3 push-ups every day. When those 3 push-ups feel easier, you could throw an extra rep in there. So now you are doing three sets of 4 push-ups every day. When the set of four gets easier, go for five. As you can see, just like with Milo, you are increasing the load on your body gradually over time. As your body gets used to the current load you're putting on it, you increase it and work at that level until your body gets used to it.

This is not dissimilar to how we learn in school. First, you learn letters, then words, then sentences. Once you have that, you can string sentences together to form paragraphs and write stories. You don't go in on day one and write a novel. You operate at a certain mental capacity and gradually increase the complexity of what you're doing. Your mind is strained at first but begins to learn; then, you strain it some more and continue learning.

Exercise Types

Now that we've covered some terminology and the idea of progressive overload, it's time we talk about some actual exercises to start building real strength. I think it's useful to group exercises into categories. This way, you only have to think about a few different categories rather than the thousands of different exercises out there. The categories I go with are:

~ Pull
~ Push
~ Hinge
~ Squat

These are the fundamental human movements, and thinking about human movement like this has really helped me think about improving my body regarding flexibility, mobility, and strength. I came across this through the work of Dan John (see appendix for more), who has had an incredible impact on my life.

Squat

Let's talk about the squat first. The best way to learn to squat is to try and emulate a two or three-year-old child. When they want to interact with something on the floor, they rarely bend over as adults usually do. They squat down. Their feet are planted flat on the ground, and they sit back with their weight spread evenly over their feet. Their knees push out to the sides a little because their hips and their body kind of slide down in between their legs.

Squatting essentially covers sitting down and standing up. Imagine sitting on a very low stool or using a toilet in certain places around the world where the toilet is a hole in the floor. When squatting, you mainly use the muscles in your legs, but a whole bunch of other muscles will be used for stability, especially when you start adding weight.

It should be pretty clear why squatting is a fundamental movement. We need to go from a sitting to a standing position. This is something that gets more difficult as we age. It's one of those uncomfortable realities that we're all aware of but might not think about. This doesn't just happen over a day, either. As we get older, it's a gradual decline. We don't see it happening, but it is happening, and there's nothing we can do about that. But you can delay it and be better prepared. Good squatting technique and strong legs will serve you well into old age.

I have found that squatting has greatly benefited me. As I described earlier in the book, there are days when standing up is painful. It makes you feel the sting of mortality and dread of life without mobility. But with the technique I've learned from squatting, I feel strong, and I can apply that technique and strength to my daily movements.

Push

The push movement can be split into two further subcategories: horizontal and vertical push. Think about pushing something away from your body. In a street fight, for example, you'll often see it begin with a push. That would be a horizontal push. For a vertical push, picture Superman rescuing a bunch of people by lifting the rubble of a collapsed building off them and over his head.

In the world of exercise, a push-up is probably the most familiar movement that would be classed as a horizontal push. An overhead press (where you press some weight from your shoulders to over your head) would be a vertical push.

These movements will primarily hit your chest, arms, and shoulders, but as with the squat, there will be a whole bunch of other muscles working to stabilise your body as you do them. In your day-to-day life, you probably won't find yourself pushing things too often. Maybe if your car breaks down, you might have to give it a push, or if your job involves a lot of manual labour. But this movement is still very valuable, especially overhead pressing. This will help create strength and stability in your shoulders – a common joint for injuries.

I also have to consider upper body strength a lot as I age. As my spine and hips degrade due to arthritis, I can compensate using my upper body. For example, pushing myself up out of a chair or, if it comes to it, leaning on a walking stick.

Pull

The pull movement is probably the most neglected movement out of the four that I have listed. Back muscles aren't considered sexy, so they don't get the same attention that a big chest or massive biceps do. But for me, the practical benefits of pull movements are immense.

Similar to the push movement, there are also vertical and horizontal versions of the pull. The exercise most associated with the vertical pull would be the pull-up or chin-up, which would be a vertical pull. This will work your arms and your back, along with various other stabilising muscles.

Pull-ups are hard, but they are worth it. What I love about pulling exercises is their impact on your posture. As mentioned before, my spine can feel like it's made of paper, so having strong muscles supporting it and keeping me upright is essential.

For the horizontal pull, imagine pulling a rope in a tug-of-war contest. You are still using your arms and your back, but you are pulling toward your chest.

Hinge

The hinge movement is probably the least intuitive of the bunch. If you've never worked out before, you could probably guess what the other three movements look like, but this one is less obvious - and it is possibly the most important. The hinge comes from bending at the hips, and believe it or not, this is the primary source of power for the strongest people on earth and provides the "snap" that allows athletes to move quickly and with power and intensity.

The exercises most commonly associated with the hinge movement are deadlifts, hip thrusts, and kettlebell swings. To deadlift, you just need to pick a weight up off the floor, but you need to do it properly. A hip thrust involves sitting with your upper back against a bench or couch with your feet flat on the floor and simply lifting your hips. A kettlebell swing involves swinging a kettlebell between your legs and up to your chest.

The main muscles behind the hinge are the glutes (your ass) and the hamstrings (back of your legs, above the knee). If you bend over to pick something up, you are hinging. As you stand up out of a chair, you will also be hinging. When a boxer throws a punch, the real power comes from their hips. The same can be said of a footballer that turns on the spot and takes off in a sprint. If you look at powerlifters, strong men/women, and Olympic weightlifters, you will often find they have big asses. Real strength is in your ass, not your biceps or your chest.

Did you know . . . The power of the hinge

In 2016 Eddie Hall broke world records and became the first man to pick 500kg up from the floor – 500kg, that's more than six of me! That was a hinge; the power to lift that weight came from his hips. The glutes and hamstrings truly are the powerhouses of the human body.

When it comes to strength and mobility, if your hip hinge isn't strong and your hips aren't mobile, you are not strong or mobile. Period. This is the movement that keeps you young. Keep these muscles strong, and your transition to old age will be as smooth as possible.

Personally, this movement is the most important to me. It was in my hips that I first felt the pain of arthritis, so I know firsthand just how limiting it can be to not have your hips on your side. Everything gets more difficult. Standing up, sitting down, walking, standing, lying down – all of it. And with reduced mobility due to hip pain, your health is guaranteed to be impacted. If you can't move, your body will start to deteriorate. If I could only focus on one movement, this would be it.

Carrying

We've all been there. You, or a parent or significant other, have just returned from the shop with a car full of bags of stuff that must be carried into the house. The idea of making multiple trips briefly crosses your mind before your ego steps in and says, *"Pft, I can carry all of that in one trip."* So you load up your arms with bags and proceed to waddle toward the house, trying to navigate the various obstacles in your way while carrying this additional weight.

Carrying is a human endeavour. Walking and carrying is what we've done for most of our existence, whether it's carrying children, the kill from a hunt, jugs of water, or foraged food. If you pick up heavy things and carry them around, your body will thank you. Not while you're doing it, of course, but afterwards. Your capacity for work will increase, your bones will get denser, and your muscles and joints will get stronger.

Walking with weight will also increase your heart rate, yielding cardiovascular benefits. So along with the fundamental movements (push, pull, hinge squat), carrying heavy things is a great thing to do.

Tonic and Phasic Muscles

I want to briefly cover a categorisation of muscles called "tonic" and "phasic". It is a useful way to think about how you work with your body as it ages.

Tonic muscles can be thought of as always being engaged. These are the muscles that are always working. For example, the muscles up and down your spine are always working to keep you upright. The same goes for the muscles in and around your stomach. The muscles at the back of your upper leg (hamstring), chest (pectorals), and biceps would also fall into this category.

Phasic muscles, on the other hand, can be thought of as our powerhouses. These muscles are generally just sitting there relaxing until we need them to do some work. Think upper back, glutes, triceps (opposite your biceps), shoulders, and quads (front of your upper leg). Often you might find these muscles weakest when you start working out. The tonic muscles are always working, so you at least have a starting point, but that's not true of your phasic muscles.

One way I've heard this explained that I found useful was to imagine you are climbing a tree, but as you reach the top, a storm comes out of nowhere. The wind begins to howl, and the tree sways violently in the gale. It's too risky to climb down, so you need to hang on. You wrap your arms and legs around the trunk and cling to it for dear life. Think about what that would feel like. Try it now. Squeeze your body as if you are clinging to a tree. The muscles you are using in that scenario are your tonic muscles. They produce the stability and rigidity you need to stay fixed to the tree.

After a short while, the wind passes, so you climb down. Once you get back to solid ground, you take a relief-laden breath. The relief passes quickly, however, because out of no-where, you are jumped by a mountain lion. This day is not going well. The lion sends you tumbling to the ground, its paws pinning you down.

At this point, your survival instincts kick in hard. You try to push the lion off you, extending your arms to maximise the distance between its teeth and your face. You kick your hips up to try and throw it off balance and take the weight of its body off yours. Your arms are now overhead, pressing against its rib cage, trying to push it onto its back. It works, giving you time to run for it, back to the tree. You jump and pull yourself up out of reach. In this terrifying struggle, your phasic muscles do most of the work. As you extend your arms and push the mountain lion away, your triceps work hard. To lift your hips and roll the mountain lion over, your glutes kick into overdrive. Jumping to your feet and pulling yourself up on a branch engages your quads and upper back.

The reason I wanted to talk about tonic and phasic muscles is that they behave a little differently as you age, so they are worth thinking about. Tonic muscles tend to shorten and get tight as we age. Phasic muscles, on the other hand, tend to weaken. If you let this happen, you will end up with the pos-ture of Mr Burns from the Simpsons. Your shortening core and chest muscles pull your shoulders forward into a hunch, and your weakening upper back muscles let it happen. Your biceps get tighter, pulling your forearms up as your weakening triceps make it harder to extend your arms. Weakening glutes and tight hamstrings tilt your pelvis, increasing pressure and risk of injury on your lower back. And finally, weakening quads make it harder to stand and sit down.

So what do we do? Well, in general, it is a good idea to stretch out your Tonic muscles, ensuring they are loose and flexible while at the same time strengthening your Phasic muscles. Really you want to strengthen them all, but stretching tonic muscles and strengthening phasic muscles is a good rule of thumb.

Did you know . . . A standing desk can improve your posture

Like many people, I spend a lot of time at a computer, and for me, sitting for long periods leads to a lot of pain, so investing in a standing desk made a lot of sense. I was expecting some difference, but I was amazed at how much of a difference it made to how I felt physically. I cannot recommend getting a standing desk enough.

Creating an Effective Workout

With all this in mind, how do you create an effective workout? It's actually pretty simple. All you need to do is select one exercise that you can do for each of the fundamental movements. For example, applying all of the information above can put together this simple workout:

Repeat three times:

- ~ 10 push-ups (push)
- ~ 10 squats (squat)
- ~ 10 hip thrusts (hinge)
- ~ 10 bent-over rows (pull)
- ~ Rest 60 seconds

If you aren't familiar with some of these exercises, don't worry about it for now. What's important is that you cover the fundamental movements without needing any equipment and could knock this routine out in about 10 minutes. Throw in a quick warm-up and a few stretches, and you'd be done in less than 20 minutes. Each of these movements can be made easier or harder, so you can start easy and make it much more difficult over time, building strength as you do.

If you did this workout every day for a week, you would see progress very quickly. There are 10,080 minutes every week. At 20 minutes each day, this routine would take 140 minutes per week. That is 1.3 per cent of your week. It's a tiny invest-ment in your body that will yield huge long-term gains.

Couple simple strength training with walking and fueling your body with good food, and you will be set for life.

The specifics aren't important right now; the point concerns the importance of strength, how everyone can get stronger, and how it's a lot easier than the fitness industry would have you believe. You just have to take some ownership of it yourself. Take control of your body and learn what it can really do.

5. Breathe

"Feelings come and go like clouds in a windy sky. Conscious breathing is my anchor."

~ Thich Nhat Hanh

Breathing for Peace and for Power

Use breathwork to your advantage

If you want to instil fear into someone, real fear and panic, take away their air. This is universal. It doesn't matter how big and strong you are; being unable to breathe causes all sorts of primitive circuits in the brain to fire up into overdrive. Once the body stops getting oxygen, everything else is immediately deprioritised, and getting oxygen becomes our sole reason for existence. Actually, it's not the lack of oxygen as much as the build of carbon dioxide. If you breathe all the way out and hold, you will find the urge to breathe seems to increase exponentially. Your body is still active while you're holding your breath out; it's still producing carbon dioxide as a waste product of that activity. As CO_2 rises, you experience more and more discomfort.

Breath and the Nervous System

Being unable to breathe is terrifying, which should be fairly obvious and intuitive. Still, considering this truth, it's surprising how little we think or talk about breathing in day-to-day life. For example, did you know that there is a big difference between mouth breathing and nose breathing?

I didn't either, but there is. The nose is actually a pretty advanced filtration and humidification system. Each breath taken through your nose is filtered by tiny hairs, eliminating pathogens, dust and pollen. That air is also humidified, meaning moisture is added to it. This prevents drying out your lungs and the various little tubes and pathways. Nose breathing also increases oxygen absorption. As I've already mentioned, your body's desire for oxygen increases as carbon dioxide increases. Breathing through your nose forces you to breathe more slowly, which allows more CO_2 to build up in your blood, which in turn increases the absorption of oxygen when you do breathe. It also reduces anxiety and stress by activating a part of your nervous system called the "parasympathetic". This is the part of your nervous system that is responsible for rest, relaxation and recovery.

Mouth breathing, on the other hand, can cause a whole host of problems and even manifest physically. Chronic mouth breathing can actually change the shape of the face, making it longer and narrower. Mouth breathers miss out on the filtration and humidification provided by the nose and nasal passage and also increase the risk of throat infection, gum disease, and bad breath. Oh, and it can also increase stress as it can trigger the "sympathetic" nervous system, where the "fight or flight" adrenalin-fuelled response to danger is activated.

I wanted to cover some of this because I think it's interesting, and I wanted to provide some context around the importance of breathing. Still, once again, I don't think it makes too much sense to focus on science and studies unless you're interested in it.

What's really important here is that there are a lot of benefits to be had from maintaining some sort of breathing routine. It's up to you to figure out what that routine looks like for you. I will provide some advice about getting started and plenty of resources to follow up on once you've experienced the benefits to be had.

Did you know . . . We rarely breathe deeply enough

Shallow breathing refers to taking shallow, quick breaths that primarily involve the chest rather than deep, diaphragmatic breaths that fully engage the abdomen. While shallow breathing is a natural response to stress or anxiety, chronic shallow breathing can negatively affect our physical and mental well-being.

One of the main issues with shallow breathing is that it limits the amount of oxygen we take in. Deep, slow breaths allow for a greater exchange of oxygen and carbon dioxide in the lungs, ensuring that our cells receive adequate oxygen. In contrast, shallow breathing restricts the flow of oxygen, leading to less efficient oxygenation of the blood. This can result in feelings of fatigue, decreased mental clarity, and reduced physical performance. Over time, inadequate oxygenation can contribute to chronic conditions such as respiratory problems, cardiovascular issues, and even increased susceptibility to infections.

Additionally, shallow breathing is closely linked to stress and anxiety. When we experience stress, our body's natural response is to activate the sympathetic nervous system, also known as the "fight-or-flight" response. This response leads to shallow, rapid breathing as the body prepares for immediate action. However, if shallow breathing becomes chronic, it can perpetuate a state of stress and anxiety. Shallow breathing signals the brain that there is a threat, triggering a cycle of heightened stress response. This can lead to increased feelings of anxiety, tension, and even panic attacks. Breathing deeply and consciously can help activate the parasympathetic nervous system, promoting relaxation, stress reduction, and a sense of calm.

Putting This Strategy into Practice

Of all the six habits or strategies, breathing is the easiest to deliberately practise, but in my experience, the hardest to stick to. The amount of internal resistance I've experienced setting aside just 5 minutes to breathe is staggering. For some reason, it's a difficult mental block to overcome, even though all I need to do is sit there and breathe for 5–10 minutes. It seems easy, but you may have to fight to maintain a regular practice here. So, if you find this hard, you are not alone. I find it much easier to do a hard session in the gym for an hour than to sit down and focus on my breath for 5 minutes. This is probably because I can feel the work in the gym immediately, but with breathwork, I think the benefits are more cumulative. You need to practice and reap the benefits over time.

Here's how you can start (Note: breathwork can be problematic for some people, especially those with chronic anxiety. If this sort of breathing exercise causes distress or panic, skip this section. You can focus on the other five strategies for now).

Sit or lies somewhere comfortable; it could be on a couch, on the floor, or on a bed; it doesn't matter as long as it's comfortable.

Close your eyes and take a few seconds just to breathe, as normal, through your nose. When you focus on breathing, you will probably panic and forget how to breathe. Don't worry about it; this is normal. Once you're comfortable and breathing normally, you're ready to start controlling your breath. You will want to try and breathe into your belly, but if you struggle with this, don't worry about it for now.

1. Breathe in through your nose for four seconds.

2. Hold for four seconds.

3. Breathe out for four seconds.

4. Hold with your breath out for four seconds.

5. Repeat.

That's it, and it's called "box breathing". Do it for 5 minutes (20 reps) and see what happens. Hopefully, you find that the beginning of the process is uncomfortable but gradually gets easier as you keep going. And hopefully, you feel calm and relaxed by the end. Over time you can increase the length of the breaths and holds. I usually breathe and hold each breath for 6–8 seconds, but it took me a while to get comfortable with going for this long.

When I'm feeling sore and or stressed (often, arthritis flare-ups come with feelings of stress, as everything just becomes that little more difficult), I use this breathwork exercise, and it really does help. I also do it first thing in the morning as part of my morning stretching routine. I'm usually pretty stiff and sore when I get up in the morning. By the end of my stretching and breathing routine, I'm good to go.

Over time your control over your breath will improve, improving your ability to use your breath for power and control. The next step in applying this is to incorporate this conscious breathing into your stretching and mobility work. Breathe in when relaxed and breathe out for effort. Breathe in to create space and breathe out to stretch. I don't really have a prescription for this; it's exploratory. Words can only do so much to guide you; you need to get stuck in and figure out yourself.

You need to learn how your body feels for yourself because you're the only one that can feel it.

Stretching and Breathwork

The core of my evening stretching routine only contains two stretches. As I do these stretches, I really focus on my breathing. It's important to stay calm and try and breathe slowly. As you breathe out, you can push yourself deeper into the stretch. I'm confident you will find more range in your stretches if you breathe consciously while doing them.

First up are the hip flexors, which get tight and shortened by sitting all day. The second is my hamstrings. So, here's what you do:

1. Kneel on the floor so that only your right knee is on the floor and your left leg is in front with your foot flat on the ground. Basically, just kneel on one knee. Your right knee to your right shoulder should be a straight line perpendicular to the ground. Your left knee should be at a right angle. If your floor is a hard surface, you'll probably want a blanket or something to kneel on.

2. Once you are set up, take a deep breath into your belly, as best you can, nice and slowly. Then, as you breathe out, move on to the next step.

3. Squeeze your glutes (ass) as much as possible and push your hips forward slightly. Don't twist or anything; your entire body should be facing straight in front of you. You should feel a stretch right where your right leg meets your hip. Lean into this stretch for 30 seconds or so, breathing slowly. Push your hips forward slightly each time you breathe out and explore how it feels.

4. Next, straighten your left leg out so that it is stretched out in front of you. Your left heel should be on the ground now, with your toes pointing at the ceiling, and you should still be sitting up tall, keeping your back straight. Again, take a big deep breath into your belly, and as you breathe out, move on to the next step.

5. Pull your toes back toward your knee. This is a small movement, but you should feel the entire back of your left leg light up. Once you feel the stretch, breathe in deep again, and exhale slowly as you move on to the next step.

6. With your back completely flat, start to lean forward. As soon as your back curves or hunches over, you have reached the limit of your flexibility here. Stop there. Feel free to hang on to a couch or a wall for balance. Keep breathing slowly and deeply.

7. Now, lean forward as far as you can without hunching over. The goal will be to get your hands flat on the floor and your belly touching the front of your leg, but that might take a few weeks (or months) of practice.

Remember to breathe. As you exhale, try to stretch deeper. As you inhale, get comfortable in the position you are in. Don't hold your breath.

Repeat on the opposite side.

Power and Breathwork

To get power from your breath, you can try a simple push-up. If you can't do a push-up, try elevating your hands. For example, place your hands on the edge of your couch or kitchen countertop. Using your breath for power looks something like this:

1. Get yourself into a push-up position. Your arms should be straight in front of you, at 90 degrees to your body, whether doing a regular push-up or with your hands on something.

2. Take a big breath, right into your belly, if you can.

3. Squeeze every muscle in your body as tight as you can. Squeeze your legs together. Squeeze your stomach around the breath you just took. Turn the inside of your elbows forward so that your shoulders get tight.

4. Once everything is tight, lower yourself into the push-up.

5. Once you reach the bottom of the push-up position, it's time to release that tension. Breathe out hard with a hissing sound as you push. Everything should still feel tight.

Try this both with and without using your breath. If you don't create that tension, do you find the movement harder? Using your breath with exercise takes control and practice, but when you get good at it, you will have much more power in your movement.

That's it for breathing. Like all the strategies in this book, this is all about practice, patience, and consistency. Think of it as exploration. It's not something you have to do; it's something you can do that might help you in ways you can't even comprehend right now. Be curious. Go see what you can do.

6. Sleep

"Sleep is the Swiss army knife of health."

~ *Matthew Walker*

Recovery Required

Heal your body through rest

Unfortunately, sleep is the area that I struggle with the most. I'm just not very good at it. I often wake up several times during the night. Sometimes it's pain related, sometimes because my cat decides 4 a.m. is the perfect time to gift me with a live mouse. However, sleep is unbelievably important for us; it's when our bodies repair, flush waste from our brains, and build muscle. Neuroscientist and sleep specialist at the University of California, Berkeley, Matt Walker, said about sleep: "The link between lack of sleep and cancer is now so strong that the World Health Organization has classified any form of nighttime shift work as a probable carcinogen."[10]

Getting Rest

The problem with arthritis and sleep is that an extended period in one position creates stiffness, and that's what sleep is – an extended period where you don't move very much. So, what tends to happen is that we naturally shift or roll over, but

---

10 The Lancet, Oncology: News. Carcinogenicity of Night Shift Work. The Lancet, Oncology, August 2019; 20(8): 1058-9. https://www.thelancet.com/journals/lanonc/article/PIIS1470-2045(19)30455-3/fulltext

those few hours of sleep have created some stiffness, so rolling over is now painful. Sometimes that pain or discomfort will be enough to wake me up, which can happen often on a typical night.

This problem is also cyclical and compounding because lack of sleep can increase pain. Patricia Parmelee, PhD, Director of the Alabama Research Institute on Aging, University of Alabama at Tuscaloosa, explains: "Studies also show that not sleeping at night exacerbates pain the next day. But there is something about sleep disruption that predisposes people with arthritis to become more disabled over time." She continues, "We really need to treat the sleep problems so they do not contribute to the progression of the disease."[11]

This isn't only true for those of us with arthritis, either. People who sleep poorly are at higher risk of cardiovascular disease, high blood pressure, and diabetes, among other chronic conditions, due to increased inflammation as a result of sleep deprivation.

This also compounds further in that when we're tired, we are more likely to make poor decisions throughout the day. It becomes increasingly difficult to decide whether to exercise or not to eat that entire packet of chocolate chip cookies. This, in turn, can leave us feeling more tired a sluggish and negatively impact sleep further, so it just spirals out of control in a negatively reinforcing feedback loop.

Interestingly, we don't know all that much about what happens to humans that have been deprived of sleep because the

11 Arthritis Foundation. Sleep and Pain. https://www.arthritis.org/ health-wellness/healthy-living/managing-pain/fatigue-sleep/sleep-and-pain

consequences are so severe that studying it is considered unethical. After just 36 hours without sleep, you will likely experience some of the following:

- Confusion and aggression

- Euphoria

- Difficulty regulating stress and emotions

- Hallucinations

After that, you risk a severe decline in mental health and even psychosis.

Good sleep is the stable foundation upon which you build healthy habits throughout the rest of your life. If you can get a reasonably good night's sleep and fit a walk into your day (which will help you sleep!), you will likely find that many other things fall into place a little easier – making better food choices, increased focus, easier to maintain healthy and positive relationships and so on.

To ensure that I maximise my chances of a good night's sleep, I practice good sleep hygiene, which basically looks something like this:

- ~ Go to bed at the same time every night (yes, this includes weekends).
- ~ Get up at the same time every day (yes, this also includes weekends).
- ~ Get out into the morning sunlight for a walk as quickly as possible.

~ No screens an hour or so before bed. I leave my phone in a different room to remove temptation.
~ No food an hour or so before bed.

This sounds simple enough but is surprisingly hard to do. There always seems to be a show on TV that you want to watch when you should be going to bed. I just do the best I can, and I find that it does help. I generally fall asleep pretty quickly – no issues there. It's staying asleep that is the challenge.

Did you know . . . *Cold showers can make you feel better and sleep better*

Whenever I talk to people about what they can do daily to feel better, the one thing that gets the most resistance is taking cold showers. Over the years, I've come to love them, though I still hate them and understand why people are so resistant to doing it. However, I guarantee you will feel great after a cold shower. It can reduce inflammation, is great for your hair and skin, and is an excellent exercise for mental toughness. For bonus points, try taking some slow breaths while under cold water.

That being said, a cold shower right before bed might not be the best idea, as it could spike hormones that seem to negatively impact sleep. So you are better off taking your cold shower early in the day, and if you must shower at night, a warm shower (not piping hot!) is preferable.

Putting This Strategy into Practice

Putting this one into practice will look very different from person to person. We all live different lives and have very different schedules, but I want to share some ideas so that you at least have a few options to try out.

If you can, get to bed and get up at the same time every day, even on weekends. Your body loves routines and has a natural one called the "circadian rhythm", which is an internal process that regulates the sleep-wake cycle and various other physiological functions. It operates on a roughly 24-hour cycle and is influenced by external triggers such as light and darkness. It also plays a part in helping to maintain the proper timing of sleep, hormone release, and other bodily processes.

Neurobiologist Andrew Huberman talks a lot about the value of getting up in the morning and getting out into the sunlight as soon as possible, which ties into this rhythm.[12] Getting out into daylight first thing in the morning causes a spike of cortisol (a hormone) in your body. Interestingly, this large spike in the morning sets a sort of timer, so roughly 16 hours later, your body is naturally ready for bed. So, you can help improve your sleep through your actions first thing in the morning.

It will also help to establish some sort of nighttime routine. Meaning: do the same thing every night before bed, and no, "looking at my phone for an hour" doesn't count as a routine. I'll share mine for inspiration:

12 Andrew Huberman. (2021, January 11). Master your sleep & Be more alert when awake | Huberman Lab Podcast #2 [Video]. YouTube. https://www.youtube.com/watch?v=nm1TxQj9IsQ

1. Stretch and breathe calmly for 10–20 minutes (usually while watching TV).

2. Tidy up a little so I don't wake up to a mess in the morning – 5 minutes.

3. Get dressed for bed (more on this below).

4. Go to the toilet.

5. Brush my teeth.

6. Wash my face with **cold** water (more on why I use cold water below).

7. Get into bed and read (avoiding anything too intense) – 10 minutes.

As soon as I start stretching, that's it. Bed is coming. It's an advance notice to my brain to start winding down. If I'm watching a movie or a TV show, I'll usually time it so that when there are about 20 minutes left, I start stretching. Everything after that point is autopilot. This routine is so deeply ingrained that I barely need to consider it. If I ever accidentally wash my face before brushing my teeth, it feels weird.

Having done this for a few years, I get about 10 minutes into my book before drifting off. I rarely lie awake in bed analysing the day's events – although I used to. But as is a common theme with everything I've talked about in this book, consistency is key. You can't expect to follow a sleep hygiene routine one night of the week and reap the benefits.

The benefits of good sleeping habits are cumulative; they build over time.

Whatever your bedtime routine looks like, there are some goals to remember. You're trying to calm your mind and avoid stimuli. This is why stretching and breathing can help the body enter a more relaxed state. You also want to spend some time in relative darkness. I read with a backlit Kindle in a room with blackout curtains. Reading helps calm my mind further, while the darkness tells the circadian part of my brain that it's time for sleep. That said, if you read on a phone or tablet, the screen provides some serious stimulus, so if you must use yours, try enabling a "blue light" filter. This will reduce the amount of blue light emitted, linked to disrupting hormones critical for helping us sleep.[13]

I've also got a few specific things you can try, though they will all require a lot of discipline.

Put Your Phone Out of Reach

Staring at a screen in bed is not a great way to end the day. First off, there's the blue light that will wake your brain up. Then there's the anxiety-inducing social media feeds we often scroll through endlessly. It's also not a great idea to start the day in this way either, and the simplest solution is simply to leave your phone in a different room.

The usual excuse for not doing this is, "I need it for the alarm." Alarms are cheap (though if you have the money to

---

13 Sleep Foundation. (2023). How blue light affects sleep. Sleep Foundation.https://www.sleepfoundation.org/bedroom-environment/blue-light

spend, I'd recommend a wake-up alarm that mimics daybreak), or just leave your phone out of reach on the other side of the room. This has the added benefit of making it harder to snooze in the morning.

Lower Your Body Temperature Before Bed

To get good sleep, the core body temperature needs to drop by 2-3 degrees Fahrenheit, and as Sleep expert Matthew Walker explains: "For you to get the heat out of the core of your body, you actually need to release that core heat through the outer perimeter surfaces of your body, namely your hands and your feet."[14]

Remember earlier in my bedtime routine how getting changed for bed came early in the sequence and that I wash my face with cold water? And that I'd explain later? Here's why. I like to walk around barefoot, helping the heat leave my body. The cold water on my face and hands helps too. I stick to this even in the dead of winter, which means ice-cold water in Ireland.

I even go one step further because I feel hot but don't like sleeping with thin sheets, I use a Chilli-pad. This material wraps around my mattress and has rubber tubes running through it. Those tubes are attached to a kind of air conditioning unit, which pumps cold water through them. This means I can precisely set the temperature for my bed. The unit was not cheap, but the benefits have been significant. There are also "cool" mattresses and "toppers" available that include

---

14 How To Sleep Better with These Bedtime Rituals. (2020, June 8). Spotify. https://open.spotify.com/episode/7x4OEfSnxub8sW1ffvcijY

a layer of gel designed to keep you cool at night, although they come with a hefty price tag.

Watch What You Eat and Drink Before Bed

Avoid caffeine after 3 or 4 p.m. (or 6 hours before bed, whenever bedtime typically is for you). Caffeine will light up your nervous system, which is why people love to drink the stuff, but it will hinder your efforts to relax before bed. Probably best to go for decaffeinated or teas from later afternoon/evening.

Alcohol can also disrupt sleep. One or two drinks may help you fall asleep, but they will reduce your sleep quality, even if you haven't had enough to feel drunk. This is because alcohol alters the production of a key sleep hormone, melatonin.

It's also a good idea to avoid eating 2–3 hours before bed, or at the very least, try to avoid eating a lot. I'm guilty of always wanting a slice of toast in the evening before bed, which is probably fine – but a load of chocolate and other sugary foods is not ideal. Incidentally, I've found that when I go to bed on a full stomach, especially if I'm feeling a bit bloated, my arthritis symptoms are always worse the following morning.

Try Some Natural Sleep Aids

Every evening I rub some magnesium oil on my legs. I often get restless legs in bed (I like to run in my sleep), but the magnesium counters that, especially on days after a heavy leg workout. You can also try drinking some chamomile tea or Valerian root. Studies have shown the benefits of Valerian root for falling asleep and improving the quality of that sleep.[15] If you enjoy baths, add a handful of Epsom salts to warm water (not hot), it is great for easing aches and pains and can help relax your body before bed.

Keep a Sleep Journal

Earlier in the book, we discussed keeping a food journal, and the idea here is the same. Write what you did during the few hours before bed, and then in the morning, give yourself a sleep rating. Take notes of any disturbances during the night. It always helps to try and find correlations between poor sleep and the things you're doing. You could start by just rating your sleep for a week. Then the following week, try to go for a 20-minute walk first thing every morning and see if the rating changes.

Move More During the Day

Nothing will get your body ready for bed like physical activity. The more you move during the day, the more likely you will feel physically tired come bedtime. Get a step counter to see how active you are. What happens if you increase that activity?

That's it for sleep. As has been the theme throughout this book – exploration is key. Find what works for you, for your body, and for your life. Be mindful of the things that help and the things that hurt your efforts to live more healthfully. And most importantly – don't neglect sleep. Along with eating, drinking, and moving, it is a critical part of nourishing your body.

15 Fernández-San-Martín MI, Masa-Font R, Palacios-Soler L, et al. Effectiveness of Valerian on Insomnia: A Meta-Analysis of Randomized Placebo-Controlled Trials. Sleep Med. 2010 Jun;11(6):505-11. doi: 10.1016/j.sleep.2009.12.009. Epub 2010 Mar 26. PMID: 20347389.

*"I said it was simple,
not easy."*

~ *Dan John*

In Closing

The key piece of wisdom I've acquired over the past 20 or so years is that it all starts with consistency – which can be a superpower and a destructive force. Consistency allows a gentle flow of water to carve through solid rock. It's how musicians master their instruments, how athletes break world records, and how poets master language. Consistency is about showing up daily, even when you don't want to, and doing the work. It's about enjoying the process and letting the results care for themselves. However, consistency can also be destructive. Consistently consuming a lot of sugar, highly processed foods, or alcohol will result in health issues. Consistent under-use of your muscles will lead to atrophy.

Think carefully about what you do consistently.

The things that are easy to do consistently are often not good for us, and the things that are hard to do consistently often are good for us . . . therein lies the challenge. But there's no progress to be made by staying in your comfort zone. If you're feeling comfortable, then you're probably not making any progress. Now, this might be fine. If you're happy with where you are, then great, enjoy the comfort. But, if your goal is to change, achieve something, learn something new, etc., then expect some discomfort. In fact, it's probably worth trying to enjoy it. That will make everything so much easier.

There's nothing new or groundbreaking in anything I've written here. I think most of it is probably fairly obvious. The real problem is that while all of this is simple to lay out and discuss, it is not easy to implement. Why? Because consistency is hard.

As I've already said, you can probably build some decent strength in about 20 minutes daily. But that's every day, for years – that's the hard part. I often tell junior software engineers: "If you want to be a great engineer, read a lot of code, write a lot of code and do it for about 10 years" (which is a line I stole from Dan John and repurposed, as is "simple but not easy").

This is why enjoying the process is so important. If you can find some joy in the day-to-day mundanity of progress, then everything becomes much easier.

Appendix

Mentors and Resources

Virtual Mentors

We all have virtual mentors these days, and I think it's important to consider carefully who you choose to be yours. Here are some of mine; they are the source material for everything you've read in this book – without them, I would not be the person I am today, so I want to share some key bits of wisdom I've picked up from each of them.

Dan John

Dan John is easily my favourite person that I don't know personally. He has been strength training for over fifty years, has written many books and articles, and has coached everyone from high school kids to elite-level athletes. He is also a religious scholar (which forced me to challenge my negative feelings toward religion) and an all-around great human being.

I've learned so much from him, and I genuinely believe I have become a better person, having discovered his work. He's a fountain of wisdom, has an infectious enthusiasm for life, and is willing to share his time and experience with anyone who asks. Dan is a true role model, and I could write a whole series of books on the wisdom I've received from Dan John, but I will pick a few of my favourite ideas and list them below:

Little and often over the long haul: This is consistency – doing a small bit of work consistently over long periods will yield results. Dan also talks about another facet of consistency that is preventative in nature. Think of the saying, "A stitch in time saves nine." For example, going to the dentist a couple of times yearly. Or performing regular maintenance on your house so that it doesn't slowly fall apart and result in huge, costly repairs (that often surface at the most inopportune times).

Eat your protein, eat your veggies, drink water, and go for a walk: Dan has often said that most people's health and fitness needs could all be solved by following this mantra, and having applied it in my life, I agree 100 per cent.

- **Don't be binary:** This one is about acknowledging that few things in life are so simple that you can put them into one category or another. Life is complicated, and most things are shades of grey, not black or white. Given his area of expertise, Dan often applies this to fitness fads. If you hear someone use language like "This is the **best** way to lose fat" or "This is the **only way** to build strength," it might be time for some scepticism. But in general, I think it's probably a good idea to be distrustful of absolute language. Words like "every", "best", and "only" are often leveraged by people looking to manipulate the more primitive parts of our brains for their own gain. These days I find myself answering most questions with "It depends . . ."

- **Work on your eulogy, not your resume:** Dan has an essay explaining that your resume is what you want to tell other people about yourself or what you want them to think about you. Your eulogy, on the other hand, is what people actually think about you, the people who you care about the most. He says, "What they will talk about is when you 'showed up,' helped out, and made a difference." The idea is that you work on your eulogy by being a good person.

- **Work, pray, rest, play:** This is all about balance. A balanced life will usually consist of all of these in equal measure. If you're not spiritual, replace prayer with meditation, breathwork, or quiet reflection and gratitude. As an exercise, think about times when you felt stressed, overwhelmed, or poorly – were these elements out of balance?

Where to find him

Website: Go to https://danjohnuniversity.com/for what I think are some of the best coaching and workout programs you will find. There is also a forum full of passionate people, including Dan himself, all willing to share their experiences and help each other.

Podcast: You will find his podcast in all the usual places you find podcasts.

Books: Dan John has written a lot of books; here are some of my favourites:

- *40 Years with a Whistle: Life Lessons from the Field of Play*
- *Can You Go? Assessments and Program Design for the Active Athlete and Everybody Else*
- *Easy Strength: How to Get a Lot Stronger Than Your Competition and Dominate in Your Sport*
- *Never Let Go: A Philosophy of Lifting, Living, and Learning*

Jocko Willink

Jocko is a retired Navy SEAL commander, leadership consultant, writer, business owner, and podcaster. He looks at life through the lens of his military experience and history, which for many, will be off-putting. However, you may be surprised to find that his message is all about taking ownership, building relationships, and being humble.

It is also worth considering that war is the environment in which every human emotion exists in its most extreme form, and so there is a lot to learn from studying the lives of the people that have been through it, both troops and civilians.

Jocko's message aligns closely with Stoicism, and so I've found it useful in my attempts to build mental and physical strength in the face of daily pain.

The wisdom I've learned from Jocko includes the following:

- **Discipline equals freedom**: This sounds very militant, but it is that same message of consistency. Jocko says that through discipline, we achieve the things we want to achieve and so gain the freedom to do what we want. For example, if you're disciplined around health and fitness, you will have freedom from lifestyle diseases.

- **Extreme ownership**: This one is the stoic message. The only thing we have real control over is our thoughts. Jocko's message encourages taking ownership and looking inward. Where could I have done better? How did my reaction make this situation worse? This isn't about beating yourself up; it's about being self-reflective, learning, and getting better.

- **GOOD**: In any tough situation, try saying "good". The idea is to reframe your thinking and look for positives. I injured my leg – good, now I can focus on building upper body strength. My flight was delayed – good, now I can get some more writing done (my flight was actually delayed today, and now I am writing this section). I have arthritis – good, facing adversity is how we get stronger.

Where to find him

The main place for all things Jocko is on this Podcast, which is called 'Jocko Podcast' and is available on all major podcast platforms.

Jocko has authored several books and, on his podcast, reads books written by others. I would recommend the following (two of his, one he strongly recommends).

- *Discipline equals freedom*

- *The Dichotomy of Leadership*

- *About Face (written by Col. David Hackworth)*

Adriene Mishler

Adrienne is the creator of Yoga with Adriene, the number one yoga channel on Youtube. I've been doing her follow-along routines for years now, and every January, I do her "30-day Yoga Journey" series, in which you do yoga every day for thirty straight days.

Wisdom I've learned from Adriene includes:

- **Find what feels good**: This one has been important for me. Sometimes I'm limited in my movements, so I find what feels good instead. Note – good doesn't mean easy. It can be hard and feel good.

- **The hardest part is just showing up**: I've heard this elsewhere too, but Adriene says it a lot. I work out with some extreme consistency, but at least 60 per cent of the time, I'm not in the mood to do it. Once I start, however, it becomes easy. And afterwards, I feel great. The act of starting is where the friction usually is. Try to commit to simply starting and go from there.

Where to find her

You can find Adriene on her YouTube channel: https://www.youtube.com/user/yogawithadriene

Resources

Below are some resources I've used over the years to learn and grow. I hope that you find the same value in them as I've found over the years.

- ~ Workouts
  - o Dan John University (subscription site with workout generator)
  - o Fitness Blender (YouTube)
  - o Athlean-X (YouTube)
  - o HASFit (YouTube)
  - o Mind Pump (paid workout program)
- ~ Strength Training
  - o Dan John (YouTube, books & Dan John University)
  - o Pavel Tsatsouline (books)
  - o Mind Pump (podcast)
- ~ Calisthenics
  - o Matt Schifferle – Red Delta Project (YouTube & books)
  - o Convict Conditioning (books)
  - o Fitnessfaqs (YouTube)
  - o CalisthenicMovement (YouTube)
- ~ Yoga
  - o Yoga with Adriene
- ~ General Health & Fitness Learning
  - o Huberman Lab (podcast)
  - o Found my Fitness (podcast)
  - o Rich Roll (podcast)
  - o Mind Pump (podcast)
  - o The Pat Flynn Show (podcast)

- ~ Books
  - o *Breath,* James Nestor
  - o *The Art of Resilience*, Ross Edgley
  - o *How to Eat*, Mark Bittman, David Katz
  - o *Lifespan,* David A. Sinclair, Matthew D. LaPlante
  - o *Stillness is the Key*; Ryan Holiday
  - o *The 4 Pillar Plan*; Dr Rangan Chatterlee
  - o *Why We Sleep*, The New Science of Sleep and Dreams; Matthew Walker
  - o *Meditations: A New Translation*, Marcus Aurelius, Gregory Hays (translator)

About the Author

Kevin Bergin is a software engineer, REPs certified personal trainer, Precision Nutrition certified nutrition coach and SMRC (Self-Management Resource Centre) certified course leader.

In 2019 Kevin was diagnosed with Psoriatic Arthritis, having spent 15 years living with unexplained pain and fatigue. During this period, he focused much of his time on learning to move and feel better in the face of this unknown source of pain. This led him on a journey of discovery where he studied human physiology, strength training, nutrition, chronic disease self-management techniques and more.

Kevin has helped design and ship multiple video games, grossing over a billion dollars. Still, his primary passion is in health and fitness and, most importantly, helping other people better understand how they can get the most out of their body, regardless of any chronic conditions that may be standing in the way.

He loves walking, training, making YouTube videos, heavy metal and 80s pop music and lives in Ireland with his wife and cat. His long-term goal is to be walking, weightlifting, helping people and still learning long into old age.

www.ingramcontent.com/pod-product-compliance
Lightning Source LLC
Chambersburg PA
CBHW060457280326
41933CB00014B/2779